I0787204

Everyone can benefit from eating well and maintaining a healthy
weight. This guide focuses on losing weight, so it's been specially
designed for adults with a body mass index (BMI) of 25 or more.
You can work out your BMI using the chart on page 07 or online
at **bhf.org.uk/bmi**
If you want and need to lose weight, then this plan is for you.

Why use this plan?

Research shows that losing weight steadily and gradually is the
safest way, and the weight is much more likely to stay off than
if you lose it quickly.

This plan is not a 'diet' – something restrictive and very short-term
which doesn't work in the real world. It's a weight loss plan for life
that will help you combine the healthiest foods into a balanced
diet that suits you.

This plan is flexible, and there are no strict rules. You won't have

to count calories, or even cut out your favourite foods. Instead
you'll use the portion size guide to help you keep to the recommended amount of calories you need.

The portion guides in section 3 show you the portion sizes of common foods, making it easy to eat well and choose a balance
of the foods you enjoy and include things like chocolate, crisps and cakes as a treat now and then.

Not only will losing weight improve your health, we hope that
meeting your weight loss goals will mean you'll feel great and get more out of life.

<u>This booklet will:</u>

- **help you identify the changes you need to make to lose weight and keep it off**

- **give you all the information you need to get the nutrients needed for good health and enjoy your** food at the same time

• support you to achieve a gradual weight loss
of 1-2 pounds (0.5 – 1 kg) a week

• give you the information you need to plan changes
you can stick to – with simple tips and easy ideas
to put it all into practice.

Changing habits takes determination. But we know
you can do it and that it will make a real difference
to your health, and your future.

Do I need to lose weight?

Medical professionals use a measurement called body mass
index (BMI), to work out which of four categories you fall into
–
underweight, ideal weight, overweight or obese. Your BMI
is calculated using your weight and height measurements.
If you're in the overweight or obese categories, you are at
increased risk of a number of health conditions, including
coronary
heart disease. By losing and maintaining a healthy weight you
can
help reduce your risk and manage some existing health
problems.

**Our online BMI calculator is a quick and easy way
to check
your BMI – go to bhf.org.uk/bmi**

- it is only for adults over 18

- it doesn't apply to pregnant women

- the thresholds for the categories differ slightly with gender
and race

- it doesn't take into account adults with a very athletic build
(e.g. professional athletes) because muscle weighs more

than fat.

Talk to your doctor or practice nurse if you have any questions about your BMI.

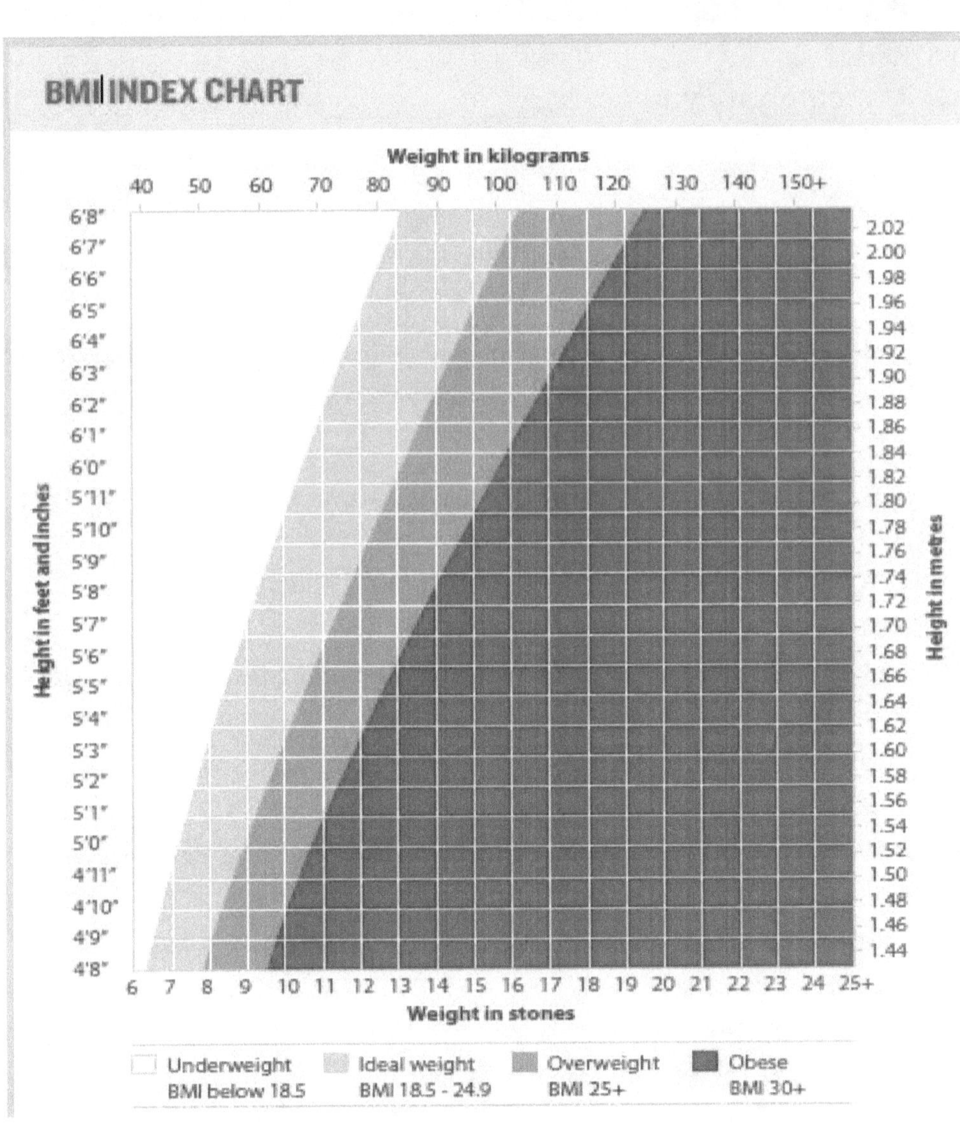

<h1 style="text-align:center"><u>To work out your BMI</u></h1>

- Find your weight across the top or bottom of the chart and then follow
the straight line up or down until you find your height on the left or right.

- Put a mark where the two lines meet and this will show you which
weight category you are in.

<u>Are you a healthy shape?</u>

As well as checking your BMI it is also important to measure your waist size. Your shape, as much as your weight, can affect
your health risk. Fat around your middle can increase your risk of
getting heart disease, cancer and type 2 diabetes. That's because
these fat cells produce toxic substances that cause damage to your body.
You can work out if you're at increased risk by simply measuring
your waist. Find the bottom of your ribs and the top of your hips,
and measure around your middle at a point mid-way between
these. For many people this will be at the level of the tummy button. Remember not to breathe in!

	Increased risk	Severe risk
Men (white European)	Over 94cm (37")	over 102cm (40")
Men (African-Caribbean, South Asian and some other minority ethnic groups)	–	over 90cm (35.5")
Women (white European)	Over 80cm (32")	over 88cm (35")
Women (African-Caribbean, South Asian and some other minority ethnic groups)	–	over 80cm (32")

'Making some changes has

helped me feel young again. I've lost 6cm off my waist and I can fit into trousers I haven't worn for years.'
Rif lost 13lb and 6cm off his waist

<u>*Your stats*</u>

Fill in your details below so you have a record of where you are starting from

Date:
My BMI:
My waist measurement:
My current weight:
My BMI category:
My risk level: (based on your waist measurement)

If your BMI and waist circumference indicate that you are overweight and/or at increased risk, don't panic – making simple
changes to your lifestyle can help you lose weight, and this plan
will support you to do that.

<u>*What weight should you aim for?*</u>

While you might have an 'ideal weight' in mind, a little goes a long

way when it comes to weight loss. Research has shown that losing
5-10% of your body weight can have big benefits in terms of your
health. It's also important to set realistic targets as you go along,
and 5-10% of your present weight is a great short-term target for
weight loss.
This doesn't mean that you can't or shouldn't lose more than 10%
of your body weight. Once you have achieved the initial weight
loss, you should look at your goals and take 10% of your new
body weight to make that your new goal. As you progress on your
weight loss journey you can continue to aim for a 10% weight loss
to achieve a healthy weight.

Target weight loss

Fill in your weight loss targets below – aiming for a 5-10%
loss over the next 3-6 months.
(To work out 5% weight loss divide your weight by 20,
to work out 10% divide it by 10)

Some benefits of 10% weight loss

• It will help lower your blood pressure and blood
cholesterol levels – which will reduce your risk of coronary
heart disease and stroke.
• You'll reduce your risk of diabetes or, if you have diabetes,

you'll be able to control it better.
• You'll become more mobile, reduce breathlessness, and there will be reduced strain on your joints which should improve any back and joint pain.
• It may help improve your fertility, and for women may reduce period pain.
• It can help improve your mood and self-esteem.

SECTION 1: GET READY TO GO

' At my heaviest I was 25 and a half
stone. I took it step by step and
I knew that unless I kept going,
I wasn't ever going to get there.'
Marchello lost 9st 7lbs

<u>*Understanding weight gain*</u>

To understand how weight gain and loss works, it can be helpful
to think about your body as a balance of energy in and energy out.
You take in energy through the calories in your food, and then you
burn this energy off through your daily routine – through things
like walking, shopping and going to work.
To stay the same weight, your energy in and energy out need to
be the same. Weight gain happens when you take in more energy
than you need.

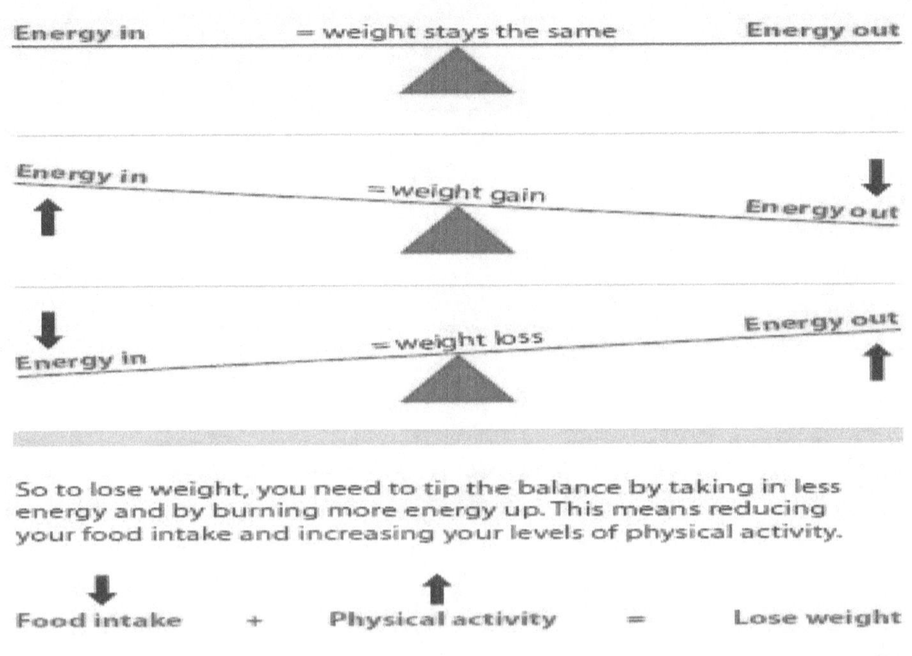

So to lose weight, you need to tip the balance by taking in less energy and by burning more energy up. This means reducing your food intake and increasing your levels of physical activity.

Before you start …

Losing weight can be hard, and managing your weight will need to
be a lifelong commitment. The habits that have led you to become
overweight took time to develop, so changing to healthier habits
will take time too.
Before you start your weight loss journey, it's important to make
sure you're feeling positive and prepared for the challenge.
Identifying things that did and didn't go well in the past can
help you plan for the future.

What factors do you think led you to gain weight?

Was your weight gain linked to a particular time in your life – for example, having children, stopping work, giving up smoking?

What do you think has helped you to lose weight in the past?

Think about the last time you were able to lose weight. What was different between then and now? For example, did you have someone to support you, were you more active, did you have less opportunity to snack between meals?

If you lost weight, then put it back on, what do you think caused you to regain weight? How quickly did the weight come back on again?

Why do you think you have found it difficult to stick to changes in your eating and activity patterns?

What have you learned from previous weight loss attempts that can help you stick with eating or activity changes this time?

Facing the challenges

It can be easy to focus on the positive things that can come from
losing weight such as buying new clothes, feeling great, and having
more energy. But often there is a cost too – to lose weight you
might need to change things that you enjoy or have been doing

for a long time, like eating less than others around you or changing
your schedule to do more activity.
Thinking about the advantages and disadvantages realistically
will help you predict the things that might make your plans difficult to stick to. This way you can think ahead and find ways
to overcome them.

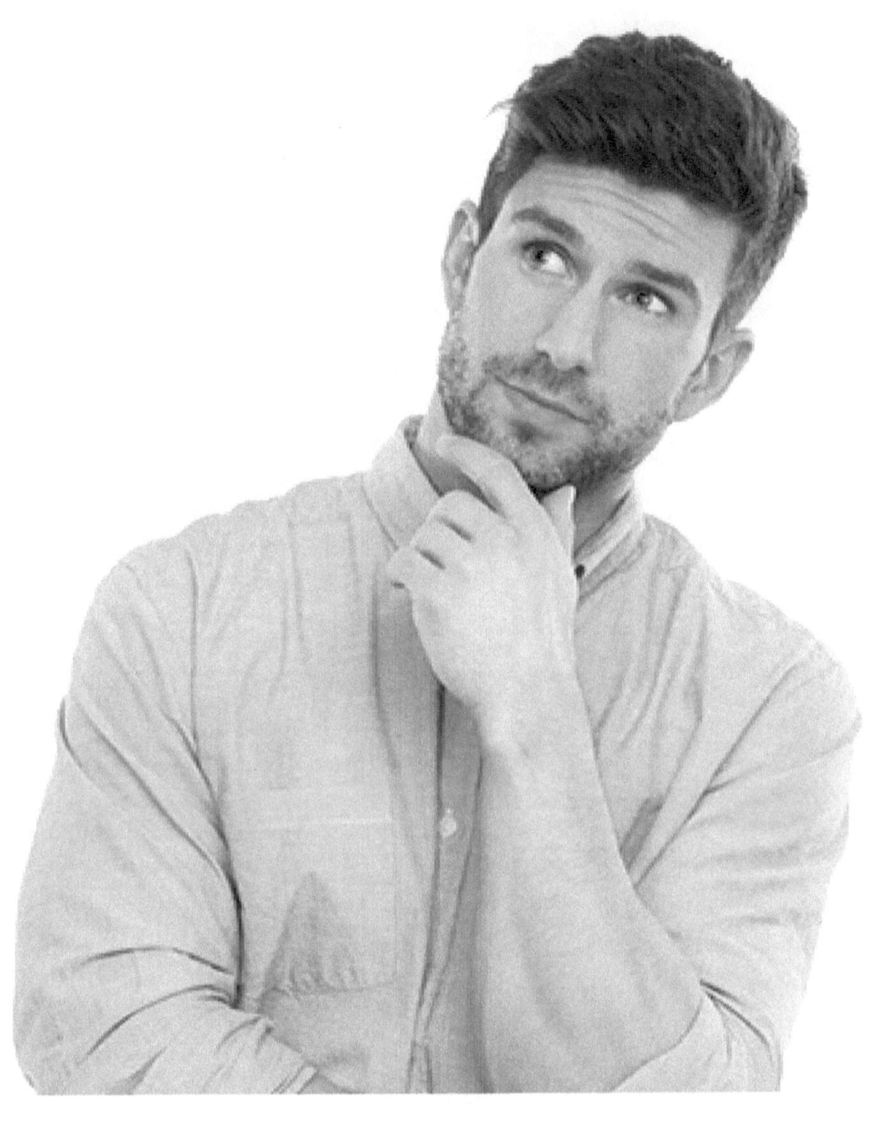

*Take some time to think about and write down the advantages
and disadvantages of making changes to your lifestyle.*

Making changes to my lifestyle	
Advantages	Disadvantages
e.g. better heart health, more energy for family life	e.g. hard work, miss out on meals out

Now think about what it would be like if you didn't change anything and stayed the same weight

Not making any changes to my lifestyle	
Advantages	Disadvantages
e.g. eat what I like, don't have to plan	e.g. putting health at risk, feel tired all the time

Hopefully the advantages of changing will outweigh the disadvantages, but think about what could help you overcome the challenges you'll face and jot down your ideas below:

How I'll overcome my challenges...

'THE HARDEST THING WAS JUST TRYING TO STAY DEDICATED – I KNEW THAT UNLESS I KEPT GOING, I WASN'T EVER GOING TO GET THERE. I TOOK IT STEP BY STEP.'

Marchello lost 9st 7lbs

Keep a food diary

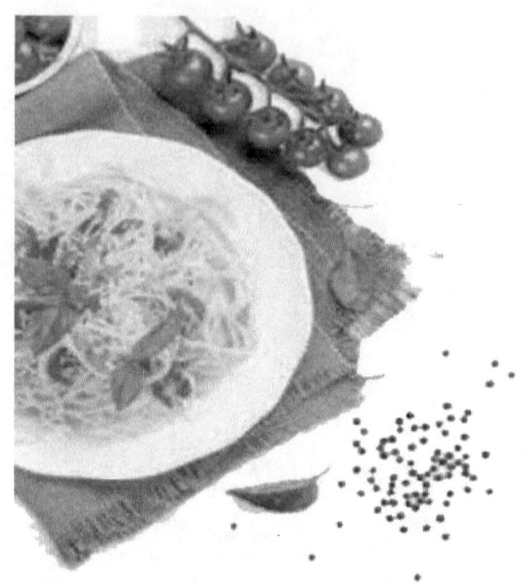

Filling out a food diary can be an extremely useful tool to help you
control your weight. The thought of writing down what you eat
may seem daunting. However, while it may be unnerving to see
everything you've eaten, facing up to reality means you've already
won half the battle.
Your food diary will help you identify what changes you need to
make to your diet and will reveal patterns in your eating that you
may not have noticed before. This can help you succeed in your
weight loss plan – for example if you can identify what times of
day you are more likely to want something to eat, you can plan
to have healthy snacks or meals on hand, or plan activities to

help distract yourself from snacking on foods high in fat or
sugar.
To keep your food diary, use the table on the following page
to
write down everything you eat and drink throughout the day.
Don't worry about what the results look like. Just be honest
with
yourself and you will be taking the first steps to losing weight
for
your health.
**For guidance on what foods fit in which groups, see
section 3.**

FOOD DIARY	Download and print out more diary sheets at bhf.org.uk/factsnotfads							
Day of the week	Meal/time of day	What I ate/drank	Fruit & veg	Starchy	Meat, fish, eggs	Milk and dairy	High in fat/sugar	Comments e.g. where I was, how I was feeling

**Set yourself SMART goals**
Once you've decided what changes you need to make to your
diet

and feel ready to make them, set yourself some goals. Goals help you
focus on making realistic changes that will make a real difference
to you. When setting your goals make sure they are S.M.A.R.T.

Specific

Be clear about the change you are making. Don't just say "I'm going to eat less" think about exactly how that will happen. Are you going to reduce your portion sizes, cut down on snacks or change what you drink?

Measurable

You should be able to measure your success. So decide how many of your snacks you are going to cut out or what you will have for breakfast each day. By making your goal measurable, you'll be able to check whether you've been successful in making the change.

Achievable

Be realistic about the changes you plan to make. You're more likely to succeed if you make small, gradual changes rather than trying to do everything at once. So start with the key areas you need to work on and build up from there.

Relevant

Make sure your goals focus on what you really need to change. Your food diary will help you pick out the most important areas to work on.

Time-specific

Write down when or how often you will make the change. Write down when you want to have achieved the change. This will make it easier for you to work out if you have achieved your goal.

SECTION 2: how the plan works
'I t's important to find ways to feel strong in yourself. Concentrate on doing it because you're the one who wants to do it.'

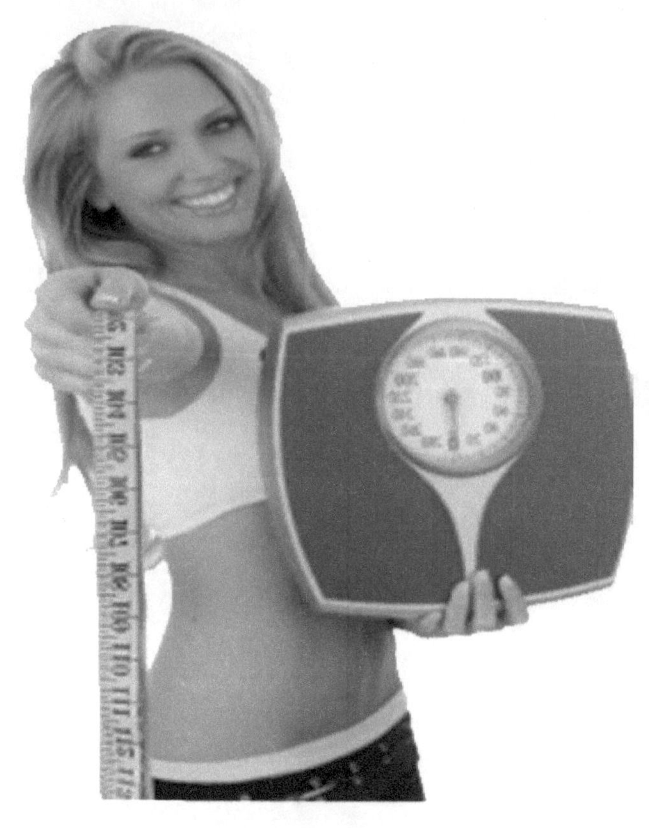

The principles of success

To help you lose weight, you need to take in less energy, and

burn more energy up. This means you need to eat fewer calories.
However, cutting down the quantity of food you eat is a difficult
change to make and doing it the wrong way – for example by skipping meals – can be bad for you.
To make it easier for you to succeed in cutting down your calories
and losing weight, there are three key areas you'll need to work on:
• getting a healthy balance of food
• cutting down on the quantity you eat
• keeping to a regular eating pattern.
By keeping to these principles and following the weight loss plan,
this should help you achieve a gradual weight loss of 1-2 pounds
(0.5-1kg) per week.
There may be some weeks when you lose more weight than this
and other weeks where your weight may stay the same or go up. There can be many reasons for this – being unwell, a special
occasion, water retention or being more active – but by tracing
everything you will be able to look back and see why this may have happened.

'I 've made changes at this time of my life and it feels great.'

**Wouldn't a diet help me lose weight quicker?**

Diets that promise quick and easy weight loss are

best avoided. You may get results fast, but they are often difficult to follow in the long term so you give up, regaining the weight as quickly as it came off. Many fad diets involve avoiding certain food groups and may not provide all the nutrients your body needs. While any weight loss will require a change to your eating habits, it shouldn't mean missing out on nutrients. Fad diets are diets that tend to:
• promise a quick, easy fix with rapid weight loss
• suggest that certain foods 'burn fat'
• promote the eating of just one or two foods
• have lots of rules about how to eat, such as the times of day you should eat
• sound too good to be true.

Getting a healthy balance of food

Eating and drinking fewer calories doesn't mean that you have to
count calories or even cut out food. Healthy eating for weight loss
means eating the right **balance** of food, but also the right **amount**
of food.
The best way to understand it is to think of foods in food groups.
We need more foods from some food groups and less from others – but you don't need to give up any single food or drink
completely. You should choose to eat mainly healthier foods that
you enjoy, but it is fine to have a treat now and again.
The eatwell plate opposite shows the types and proportion of foods you need to eat to achieve a well-balanced and healthy diet.

It covers everything you eat during the day including snacks.
For a balanced diet you should try to eat:
• plenty of fruit and vegetables
• plenty of bread, rice, potatoes, pasta and other starchy foods
–
choose wholegrain varieties whenever you can
• some milk and dairy foods
• some meat, fish, eggs, beans and other non-dairy sources
of protein
• just a small amount of foods and drinks high in fat and/or
sugar.
You don't always need to get the balance perfect at every
meal,
but try to get it right over a longer time such as a whole day
or
week and try to choose foods that are lower in fat, salt and
sugar
when you can.
Eating with the proportions of the eatwell plate in mind will
ensure you get the right balance of vitamins and minerals as
well
as starch and fibre, while keeping fat and sugar down. This
will not
only help you keep your weight down, but also reduce your
risk
of coronary heart disease, some cancers, and dental
problems.

Use the eatwell plate to help you get the balance right. It shows
how much of what you eat should come from each food group.

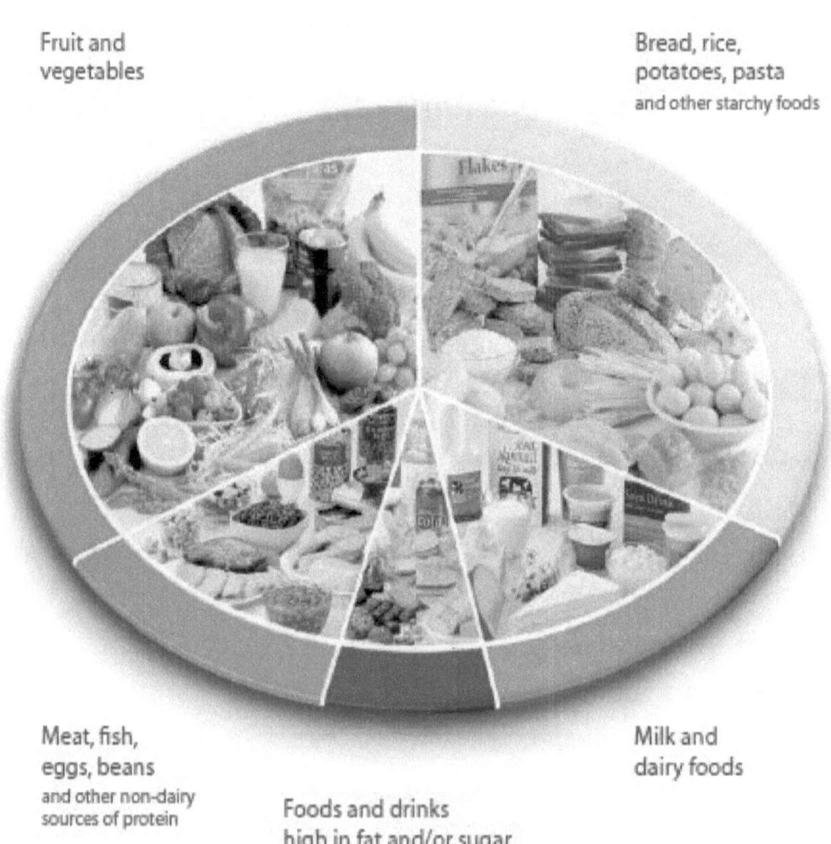

Even if you think you are already eating very healthily, it may be
that your portions are too large, which means you will be taking
in more calories than you are using up, resulting in weight gain.
This weight loss plan will help you manage the quantity, as well
as the type of food that you eat
Everyone is different, but to keep their weight the same most adult
men need around 2,500 kilocalories (kcal) a day, and most adult
women need around 2,000 kcal a day.
National guidelines recommend that for sustainable weight loss,
a reduction in calorie intake of about 500-600 kcal a day should
be combined with stepping up your physical activity levels.
To lose weight, the average man can eat or drink 1,800 kcal

**a day. The average woman can eat or drink 1,500 kcal a day
to lose weight.**
Your calorie intake includes all your food and drink and should be
based on the food groups from the eatwell plate. This weight loss
plan will help you achieve the right number of calories a day by
eating a certain number of portions of different types of food.

<u>**How many calories should I be eating?**</u>

If you normally eat a lot more than the recommended amount of
calories you may find it hard to cut back to our suggested calorie
limit and number of portions straight away.
You can use your food diary on page 22 to work out how many
portions from each food group you are currently having. If you're
eating many more than the recommended number of portions,
aim to gradually reduce your portion sizes to those recommended
in the plan, over a few weeks. If you have any questions about
the number of portions or calories you should be eating, talk
to a healthcare professional such as your GP, nurse or
dietitian.

Know your portions
How much is a portion?

With this weight loss plan, you won't have to count calories or
weigh out your food. Instead, you just need to use the portion
guides in section 3. This shows portions of common foods from
all the food groups, so you can just choose as you wish.
Portions are a funny thing. The normal helping of food you have
in a meal may contain more than one portion. For example,
a sandwich made up of two slices of bread would count towards
2 portions from the 'bread, rice, potatoes, and other starchy foods'
group and a bowl of rice may be 2-3 portions.
**You'll find guidance on portions of lots of common
foods in section 3 of the plan.**

Can I indulge ?

Nothing is banned, but foods from the foods and drinks high
in

fat and sugar group provide a lot of calories with little nutritional
benefit, so you shouldn't eat too much of foods from this group.
Think of these as foods to be enjoyed occasionally, rather than
as everyday necessities.
Although there is a limit to the amount of foods in this group you
can have each day, you can save your allowance up over the week
if you'd prefer – having none on one day and more on another.
Many people find they eat differently at weekends or when eating
out, so this way you can keep your indulgences 'up your sleeve'
for those times when you really need them!

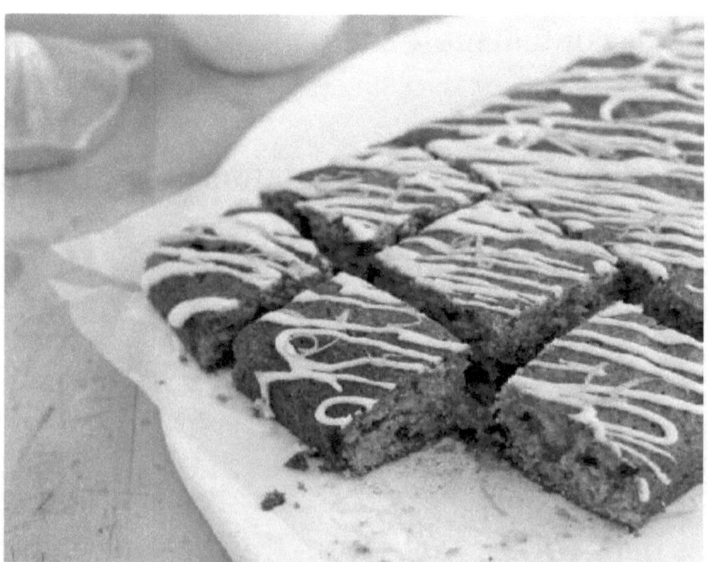

Keeping to a regular eating pattern

Eating regularly can help you achieve your weight loss goals

because it helps to ensure you don't get too hungry, meaning you'll be less likely to think about food between meals and less
likely to turn to eating high calorie snacks.
Once you get in the habit of eating at roughly the same times each day it will make it easier to control how much you eat.

What is my current eating pattern?

You can use your food diary to help identify what your eating patterns are like and ticking the boxes that apply to you below
will also help:

I skip breakfast more than once a week	
I have a large lunch and skip dinner	
I regularly miss meals and snack throughout the day	
I have a late breakfast, skip lunch and have a large evening meal	
I don't eat all day and have a large evening meal	

If you are already eating regularly then move on to the next section.
If you have ticked one or more of the boxes above, then you need
to set some goals so that you can try and eat more regularly.
Beginning the day with a healthy breakfast would be a good start.
People who eat breakfast regularly – on at least four or more days
a week – are more likely to stay a healthy weight than people who
don't. It doesn't need to be a cooked breakfast – a drink and a piece

of fruit or a pot of yoghurt is a good start to get you into the habit.

Healthy breakfast ideas include :

• wholegrain breakfast cereals like porridge with
low fat milk or yoghurt
• toast with boiled, scrambled or poached eggs
• toast with baked beans, tinned tomatoes
or grilled mushroom
• bowl of mixed fresh fruit with yoghurt
• you can have breakfast on the go too – small boxes
of wholegrain cereal, tubes of low fat yoghurt and
fruit can fit in a bag or briefcase.

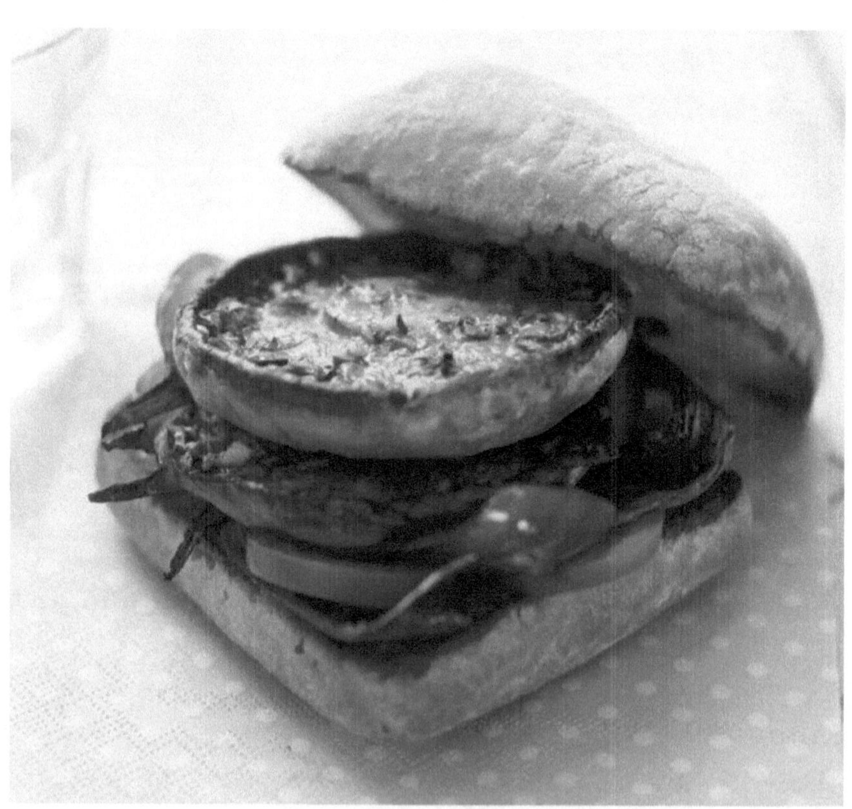

SECTION 3: *YOUR WEIGHT LOSS PLAN*

'I 've lost just under a stone and 6cm from my waistline so far. I was always making excuses – but you can make time, you've got to put the effort in.'
Rif lost 13lbs

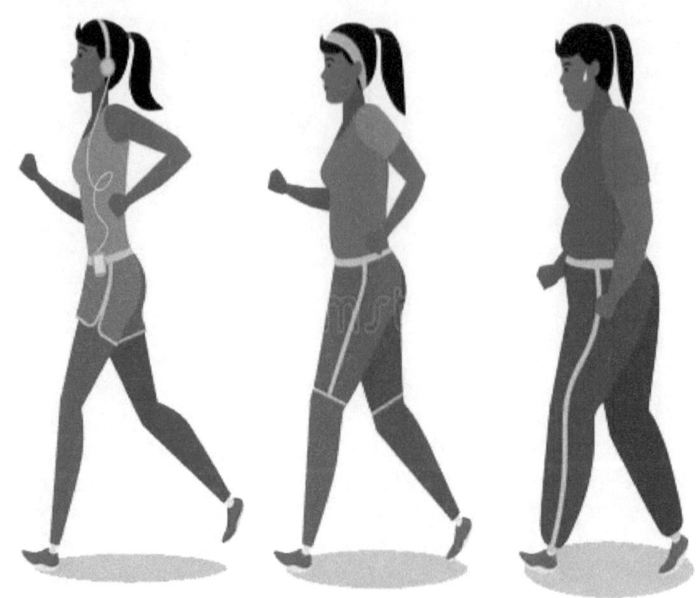

Fruit and vegetables

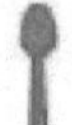
Eat 5 or more portions a day

About a third of the food you eat should be made up of fruit and vegetables. You should aim to have at least 5 portions of fruit and veg every day.
Research shows that people who eat more than 5 portions of fruit

and vegetables a day have a lower risk of coronary heart disease.
Fruit and vegetables contain vitamins and minerals which your
body needs to keep healthy and they are naturally low in fat.
They are also a good source of fibre, which makes them filling
to eat, and they will keep your digestive system healthy.
There are five ways to get your '5 a day' – the fruit or
vegetables can be:
• fresh
• frozen
• dried
• juiced or
• tinned – make sure fruit is in water or natural juice, and vegetables
are in water without sugar or salt added where possible.

Ideas to help you get your 5 a day

- add fresh or dried fruit to your breakfast

- have fruit as a snack between meals

- have a bowl of salad with your meal – if you have a ready meal, always add extra vegetables or salad to it

- add tinned beans such as red kidney beans and chickpeas to soups, stews, curry and pasta sauces

- use leftover vegetables to make soup.

<u>*A few things to remember:*</u>

*Potatoes, yams and plantain don't count towards your
'5 a day '– they are starchy foods (see page 50).

* Fruit juice and smoothies are nourishing but quite concentrated
in calories. Keep to only one portion – a small glass – of
unsweetened fruit juice or pure fruit smoothie a day. Avoid
sugary squash or fruit juice drinks which have added sugar.
* Dried fruits are quite concentrated in natural sugar so have
only one portion of these a day.

* Only one portion of pulses like kidney beans, chickpeas and
baked beans can be counted as fruit and veg. Any more portions
should be counted as a starchy food (see page 51).
*The fruit and veg in sauces, soups, puddings and yoghurts can
count towards your five a day – but watch out for the salt and
saturated fat in these foods.

* Avocado pears are high in healthy fats, but this means they are
also high in calories. Have as a salad garnish only once a week
and half an avocado occasionally as a treat

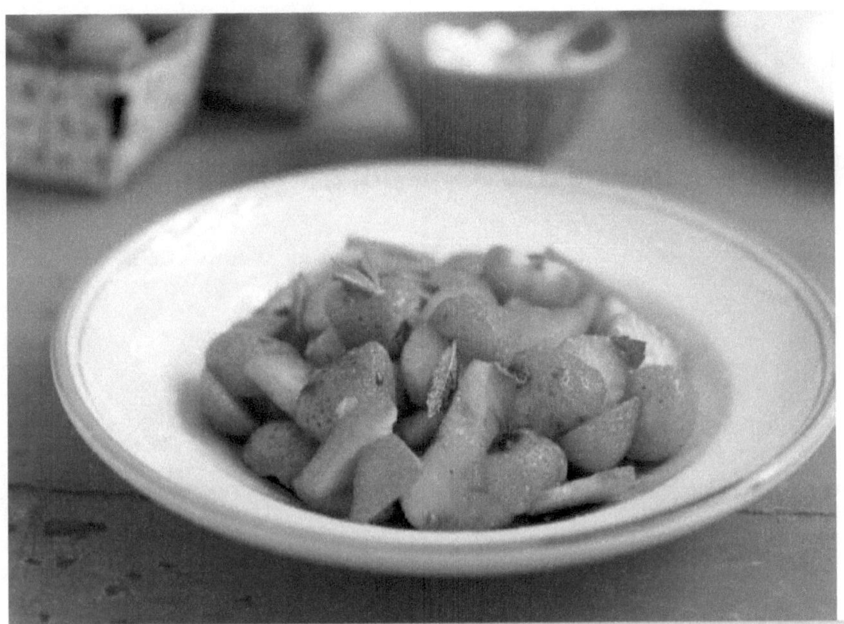

GETTING YOUR 5 A DAY

Tips and tricks to help you overcome the common challenges of getting your 5 a day:

Fruit and vegetables are too expensive	• Try buying fresh fruit and veg when they're in season – they're usually cheaper. • Buy loose fruit and veg rather than pre-packed so you just buy what you need. • Opt for the supermarket's own-brand tinned, dried and frozen fruit and vegetables – including pulses and beans – to keep costs down.
I've got no time to shop for fresh fruit and veg	• Stock up on tinned and frozen fruit and vegetables so you always have them ready to use. • Dried fruit also keeps well and you can eat it as a snack or add to cereal and other recipes.
My family don't like the taste of fruit and veg	• Set them the challenge of trying one new fruit or vegetable a week until you find some they enjoy. • Sneak in added veg to family meals – add grated carrot, chopped peppers or sweetcorn to your meals such as stirfrys, stews and even pizzas. Puree them for sauces or soups or mash into potatoes. • Cutting fruit and vegetables into easy-to-eat chunks and sticks often makes them more appealing than a whole piece – or try a fruit kebab for dessert.

<u>**Fruit and vegetable portions**</u>
Eat 5 or more portions a day. One portion is:

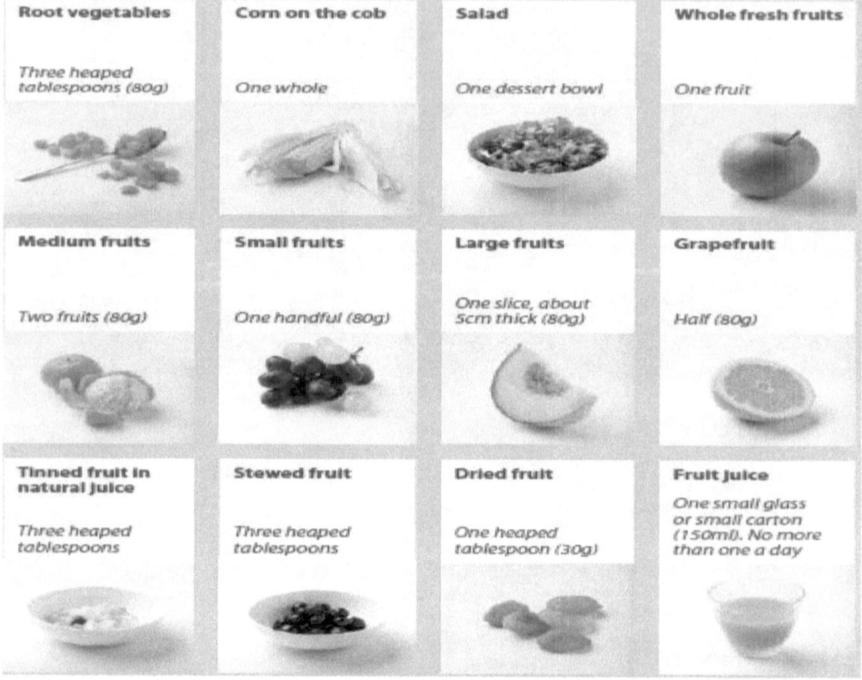

‘O ne thing I learned
was you have to plan
because it makes
life a lot easier.
If you know what
you’re preparing
you’ve got the stuff
there and ready
for you.’

Rif lost 13lbs

Bread, rice, potatoes , pasta and other starchy foods

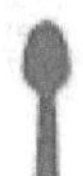 **Eat 7-8 portions a day depending on your weight loss plan**

About a third of your food should be starchy foods – this food group is our body's main source of energy and should be a part
of all meals.
Choose higher fibre/wholegrain options when possible – they contain more fibre, vitamins and minerals and provide energy that
is released slowly, making you feel fuller for longer and less likely
to snack between meals.
These may seem like small portions but remember you can use
more than one of your portions per meal (see example meal plan
on page 73).
For things like cereal, rice and pasta it may be useful to weigh

the portion out once to see what it looks like on the plate as
a guide for the future. This can also help you prepare to judge
your portions when you're eating out.

Starchy food portions

Eat 7-8 portions a day depending on your plan. One portion is:

Muesli Not crunchy *Two tablespoons (20g)*	**Muesli** Crunchy oat / granola *One tablespoon (20g)*	**Weetabix** *One biscuit*	**Shredded wheat** *One biscuit*
Bread or toast *One slice, medium thickness*	**Bread bun or roll** *Half a large bun / roll (30g)*	**Pitta bread** *Half a pitta or one mini*	**Chapatti** *One small*
Crumpet/pikelet *One*	**English muffin** *Half a whole*	**Malt loaf** *One small slice (35g)*	**Crackers** *Three*
Crispbreads *Four*	**Oats** *Three tablespoons (20g) uncooked, (40g) cooked*	**Yam** Boiled *Two egg-sized pieces or a 11/2-inch thick slice (60g) cooked*	

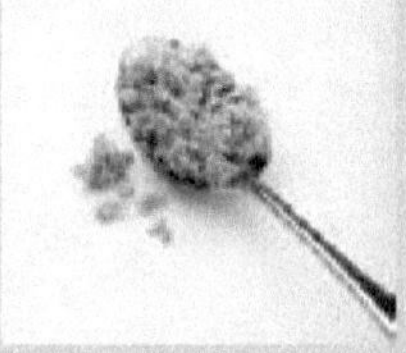

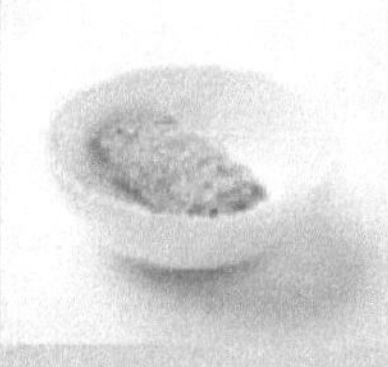

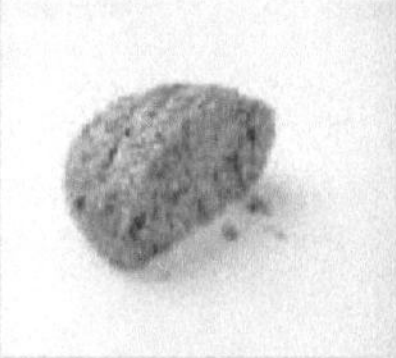

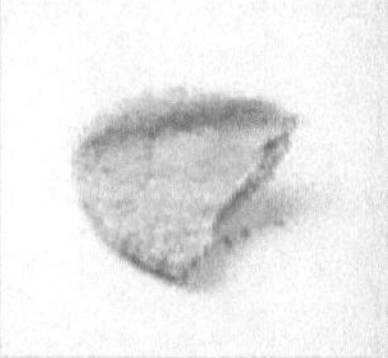

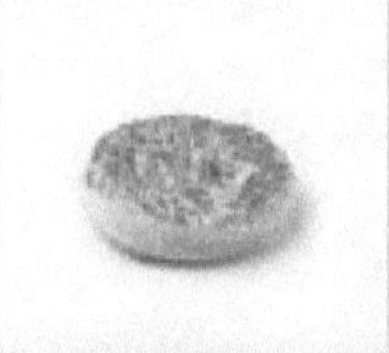

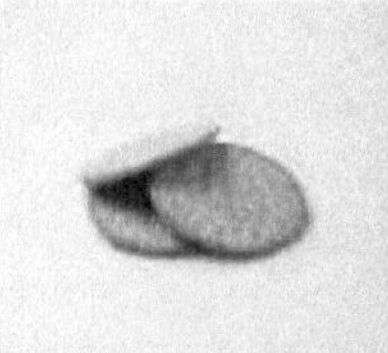

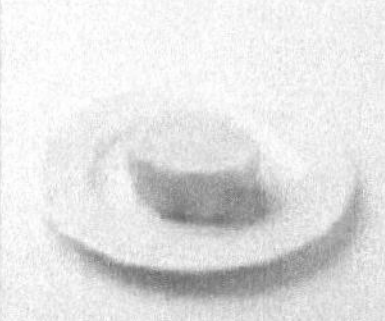

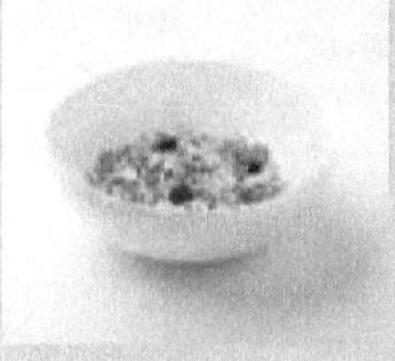

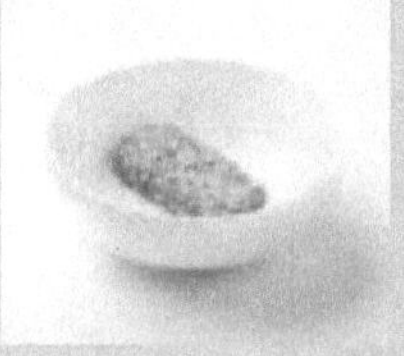

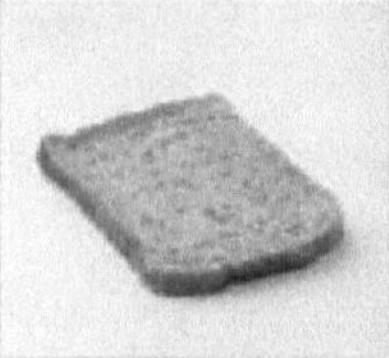

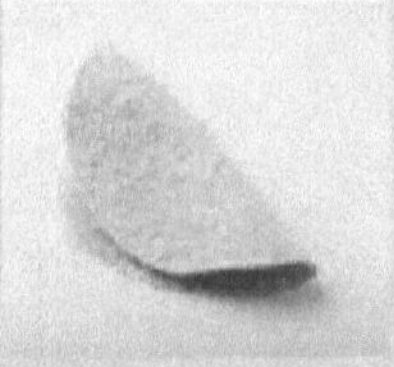

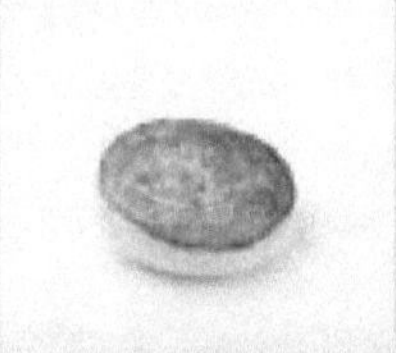

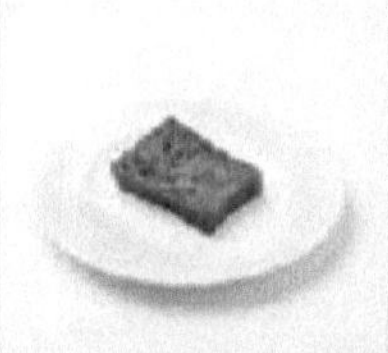

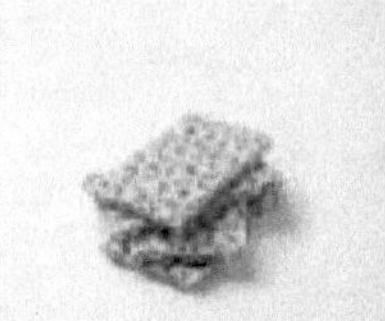

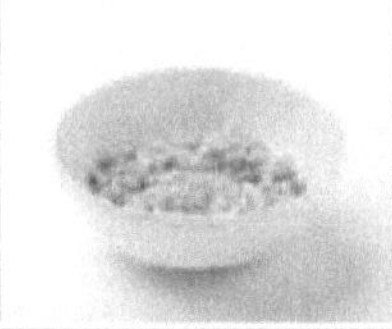

Rice	**Couscous**	**Quinoa**	**Breakfast cereal**
Two heaped tablespoons of plain boiled rice (80g)	*Two tablespoons of plain cooked couscous (40g)*	*Two heaped tablespoons of plain cooked quinoa (80g)*	e.g. flakes, crispies, porridge oats *Three tablespoons (20g)*
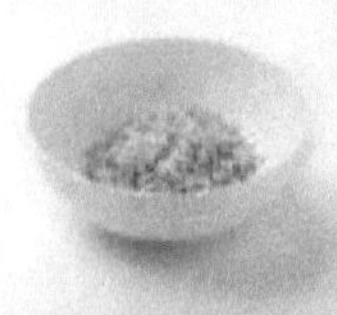	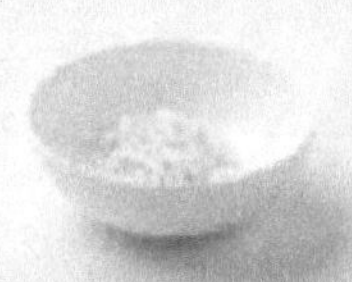	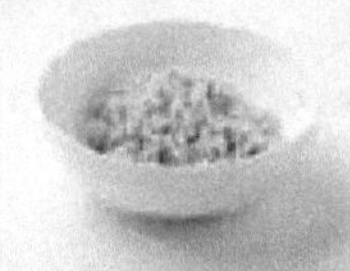	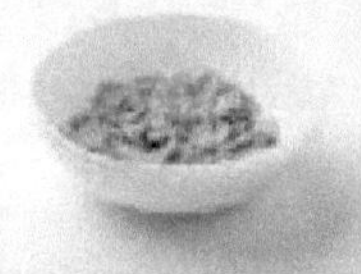
Wrap *Half*	**Egg noodles** *Half individual dry serving (25g). Three heaped tablespoons of cooked (80g)*	**Potatoes** *Two egg-sized*	**Plantain** Steamed *One medium-sized*
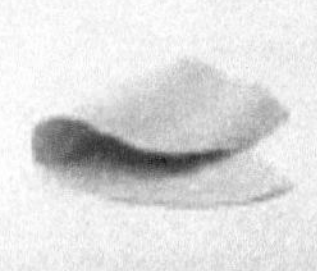	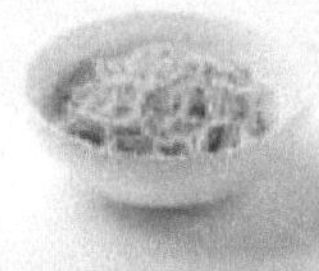	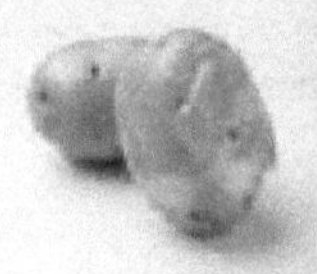	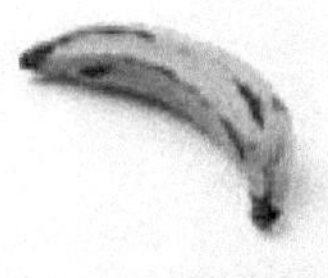

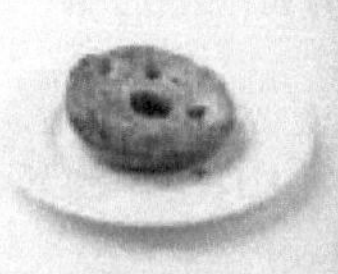

Bagel, plain or cinnamon and raisin

Half

Pasta

Three heaped tablespoons of plain boiled pasta (80g)

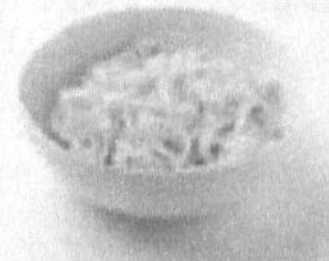

Ideas for getting the most from your starchy foods:

- Bake, boil or steam starchy foods, rather than frying them. And avoid adding fat once they're cooked – for example don't add butter to potatoes or chappatis, or creamy sauces to pasta or rice.

- Try making your own breads, rolls, scones or chappatis with wholemeal flour

- Eat potatoes with their skins on to get an extra boost of fibre, vitamins and minerals

- Add pulses such as lentils, beans and chickpeas to stews or curries

Milk and dairy foods

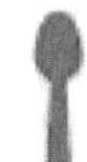 Eat 3 portions a day

This food group includes milk and milk products such as cheese,
yoghurt and fromage frais – but not butter, margarine or cream,
which are part of the food and drinks high in fat and sugar group.
Milk and dairy foods are an important source of calcium and protein.
The fat content varies a lot between different foods in this group.
Choose lower-fat versions when you can – this will mean you can
benefit from their protein, calcium and other nutrients, but have
less fat to go with it.
If you don't drink milk or eat dairy foods, it's good to use a
milk substitute like soya milk, with added calcium – go for the
unsweetened versions.

Milk and dairy portions

Have 3 portions a day. One portion is:

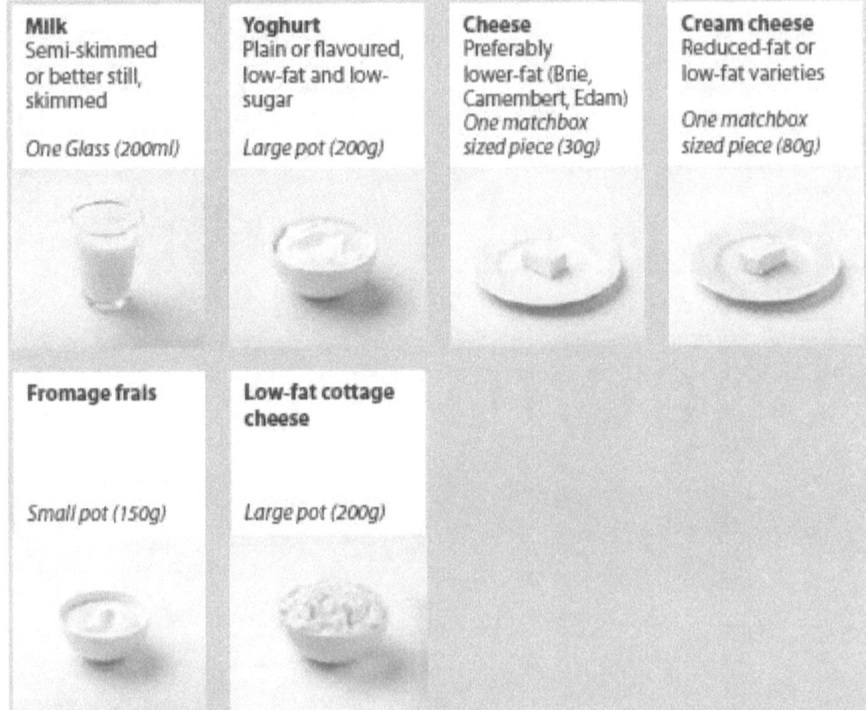

'I have skimmed milk now. I think it tastes really good.

If I have semi skimmed it tastes strange to me – too creamy!'

Vivinne lost 2st

Choosing low -fat milk and dairy foods

Check out the tables below to see how different cheese, creams
and yoghurts compare – choose the versions that are lower in fat
and calories as much as possible.

Cheese facts			
Type of cheese	Total fat per 100g	Saturated fat per 100g	Calories (kcal) per 100g
High fat (more than 17.5g per 100g)			
Mascarpone	44	29	428
Stilton	35	23	410
Cheddar, Red Leicester, Double Gloucester and other hard cheeses	35	22	411
Parmesan	30	19	452
Brie	29	18	343
Soft goat's cheese	26	18	320
Edam	26	16	341
Processed cheese e.g. cheese slices, cheese strings	24	14	297
Camembert	23	14	290
Feta	20	14	250
Mozzarella	20	14	257
Medium fat (3.1g – 17.5g per 100g)			
Half-fat cheddar	16	10	273
Reduced-fat processed cheese	13	8	228
Ricotta	8	5	144
Cottage cheese (plain or with additions e.g. pineapple)	4	2	101

Low fat (3g or less per 100g)

Reduced-fat cottage cheese (plain)	2	1	79
Quark	0.2	0.1	74

Cream comparisons

Compared item	Total fat per 100g	Saturated fat per 100g	Calories (kcal) per 100g
Cream			
Clotted	64	40	586
Double cream	54	33	496
Whipping cream	40	25	381
Double cream alternative (buttermilk & vegetable oil blend)	36	25	350
Soured cream	20	13	205
Single cream	19	12	193
Half cream	14	9	148
Single cream alternative (buttermilk & vegetable oil blend)	13	8	148
Crème fraîche			
Standard crème fraîche	31	22	378
Half fat crème fraîche	15	10	162
Fromage frais			
Natural creamy	8	6	113
Virtually fat free	0.1	0.1	49
Yoghurt			

Greek style	10	7	133
Thick and creamy	6	4	106
Greek style (sheep's milk)	6	4	92
Whole milk	3	2	79
Soya alternatives	2	0.3	72
Greek style 0% fat	0	0	57
Low fat yoghurt	1	0.7	56
Diet yoghurt	Trace	Trace	54

Meat , fish, eggs , beans and other non-dairy sources of protein

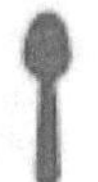

Eat 2 or 3 portions a day depending on your weight loss plan

You should eat foods that provide you with protein two or three
time a day. Protein is important for your body to work properly
and these foods will provide you with vitamins, such as B12,
and minerals including iron and zinc.
As well as meat and fish, choose 'alternatives' such as eggs, nuts
and nut butter, pulses such as peas, beans and lentils and seeds,
quorn™ and tofu.

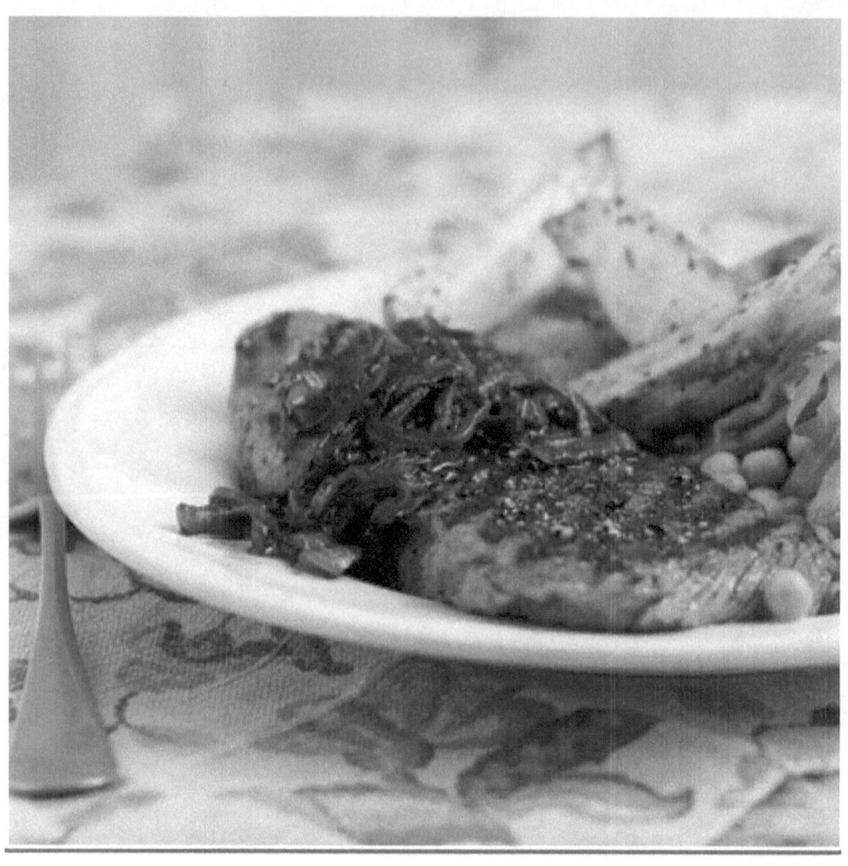

Protein portions

Eat 2 or 3 portions a day depending on your plan. One portion is:

Cooked lean meat (without skin & all visible fat removed). *Piece about the size of a pack of cards (60g-90g)*	**Fish** White *One medium fillet (150g raw)*	**Fish** Oily *One medium fillet (140g raw)*	**Fish fingers** *Three*
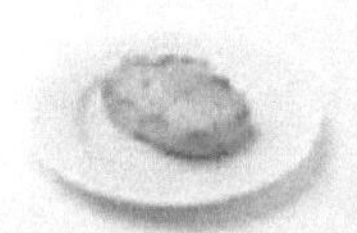	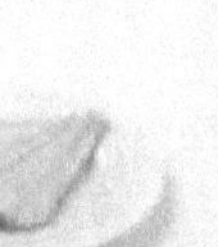	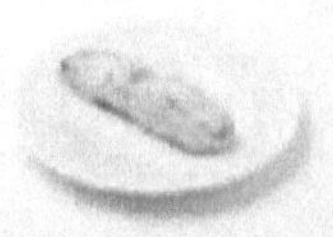	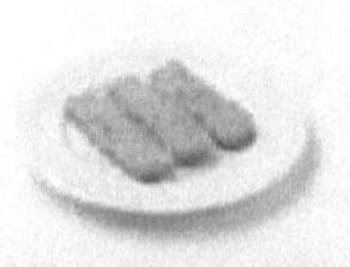
Baked beans in tomato sauce (low-sugar and low-salt if possible) *One small tin (200g)*	**Lentils** *Five tablespoons, cooked*	**Beans** e.g. red kidney beans, butter beans, chick peas *Five tablespoons, cooked (140g)*	**Peanut butter** (unsalted) *Two level tablespoons*
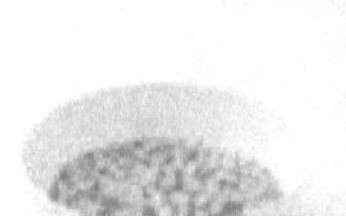	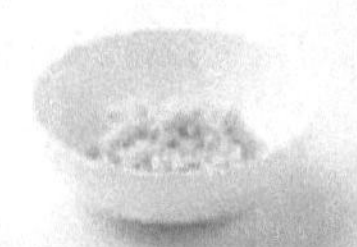	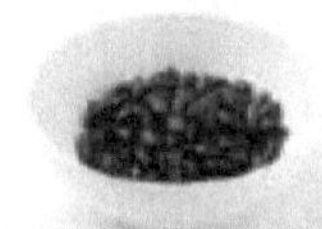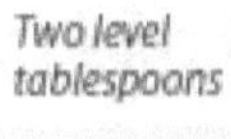	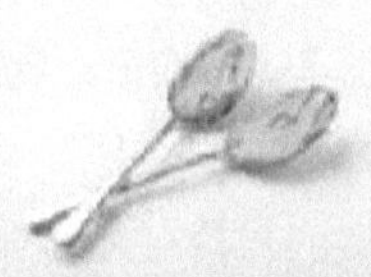
Quorn™, tofu or soya *Two sausages or 120g (uncooked weight)*	**Eggs** *Two*	**Nuts** (unsalted) *Two level tablespoons*	
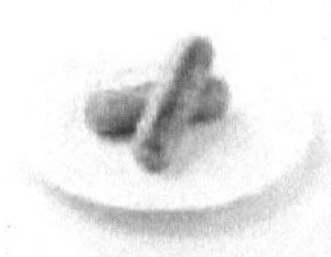	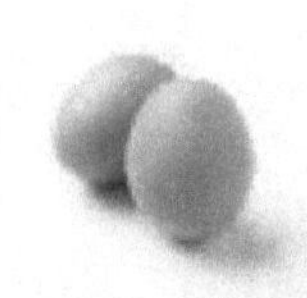	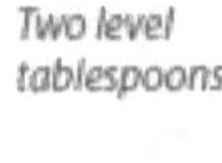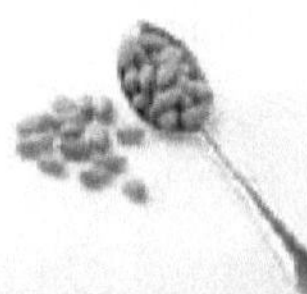	

Myth buster: Is there a limit to how many eggs you can eat in a week?

There's no recommended limit on how many eggs you should eat. Eggs can be included in a healthy, balanced diet, but remember that it's a good idea to eat as varied a diet as possible and to use healthier cooking methods when you do have eggs. Boil or poach them rather than frying and avoid adding butter to scrambled eggs.

Choosing protein foods

Some protein foods may also be high in fat, so choosing
lower fat alternatives can make sure you are getting
enough protein without that extra fat and calories.

* Choose lean cuts of meat.
* Remove visible fat and skin from meat and poultry.
* Limit how often you choose processed meats such as burgers,
bacon, sausages, and pies – they often contain a lot of hidden
fat and salt.
• Choose fish, eggs, quorn™, beans and lentils a few times a
week.
• Cook without adding fat – bake, steam, grill, poach or
microwave.

Better meat choices

The type of meat you use and the way you cook it can make a
big
difference to the amount of calories and saturated fat you eat.
Use the table below to choose meat that is better for you:

Type of meat	Higher calories & fat	Lower calories & fat
Pork	**Cooked pork belly joint with fat** Per 100g: 293 kcal 23.4g total fat, 8.2g saturated fat	**Cooked lean pork leg joint** Per 100g: 182 kcal 5.5g total fat, 1.9g saturated fat
Beef	**Fried rump steak with fat** Per 100g: 228 kcal 12.7g total fat, 4.9g saturated fat	**Grilled lean rump steak** Per 100g: 177 kcal 5.9g total fat, 2.5g saturated fat
Poultry	**Fried chicken breast in breadcrumbs** Per 100g: 242 kcal 12.7g total fat, 2.1g saturated fat	**Grilled chicken breast without skin** Per 100g: 148 kcal 2.2g total fat, 0.6g saturated fat

Spreading fats , oils, dressings and sauces

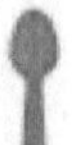 # Eat up to 2 or 3 portions a day

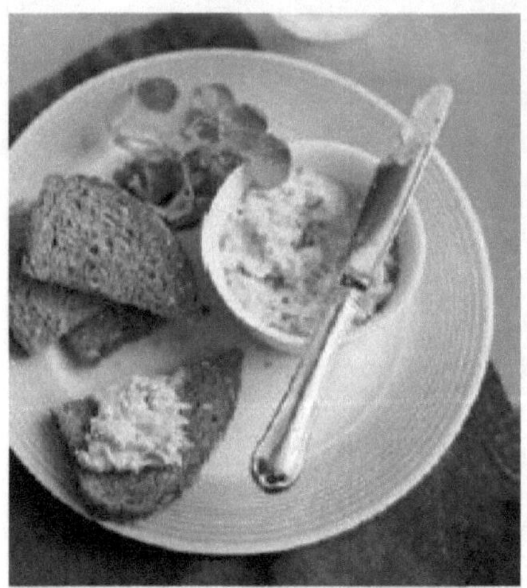

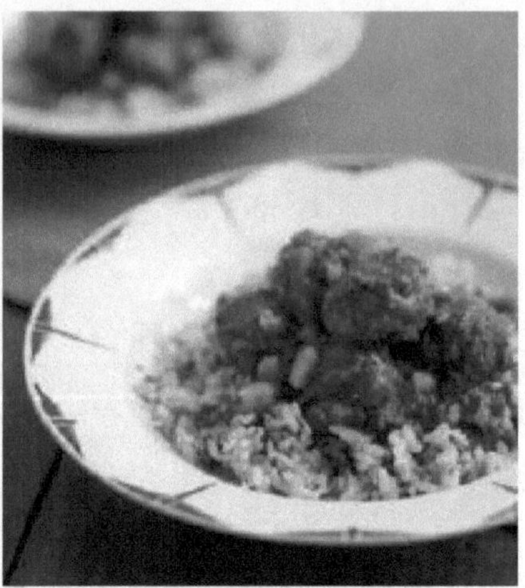

Low-fat spread	Oil (unsaturated oils, e.g. olive, rapeseed, sunflower, corn)	Butter or margarine spread or ghee	Mayonnaise
Two teaspoons	*One teaspoon*	*One teaspoon*	*One teaspoon*
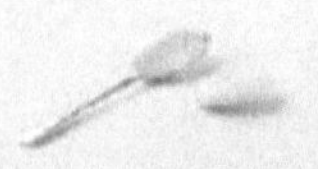	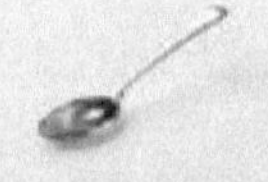	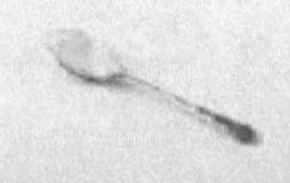	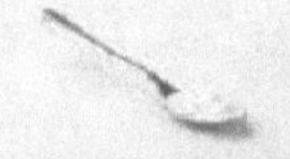

Blue cheese dressing	Salad cream	Gravy or white sauce made with fat and flour base (roux)	Gravy or white sauce (made with cornflour, no fat added)
One teaspoon	*One tablespoon*	*Two tablespoons*	*Four tablespoons*
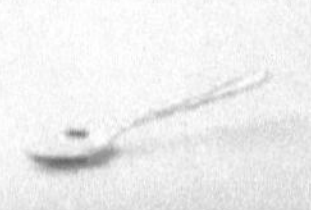	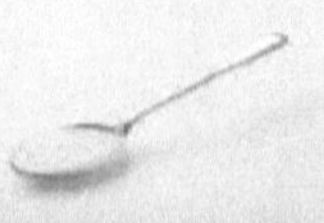	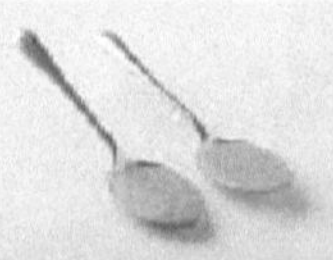	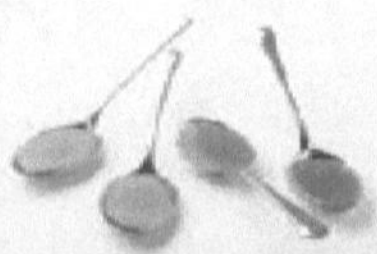

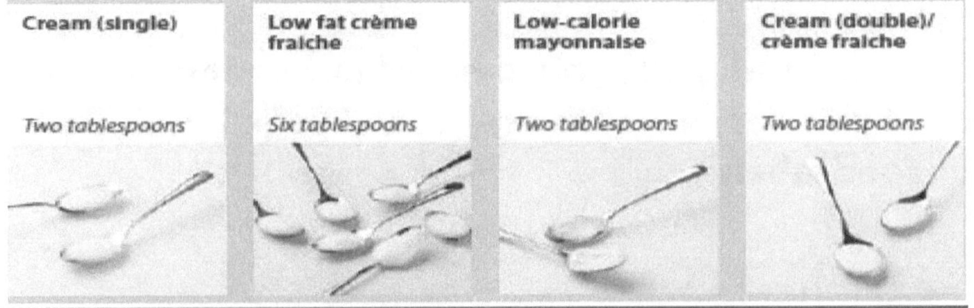

Foods and drinks high in fat and sugar

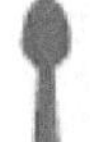 You can have up to l00kcal to 200kcal a day depending on your weight loss plan.

Remember – if you like, you can spread this allowance out over the week, having none on one day and more on another.

This group includes cakes, crisps, sweets, chocolate, sugary fizzy
drinks and alcohol. These tend to be the foods we need to cut down on. While they can be included in a balanced diet, they are
not essential.
You should aim to have only small amounts of foods in this group – swap these for healthier versions or keep them for special
occasions only.
If the foods you like aren't on the list, use the calorie information,
per serving size, from the nutritional information on the packets
to work out how much of the food you can eat according to your

weight loss plan.
Use food labels to guide you to healthier versions of these foods or healthier alternatives – look at page 79 for more info on food labels.

FOODS AND DRINKS HIGH IN FAT AND SUGAR

You can have up to 100 kcal to 200 kcal a day depending on your weight loss plan.

Sugar One teaspoon 16 kcal 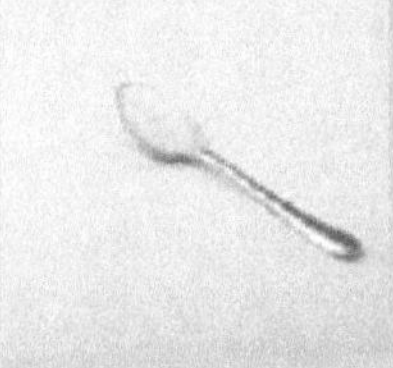	**Jam** One teaspoon 25 kcal 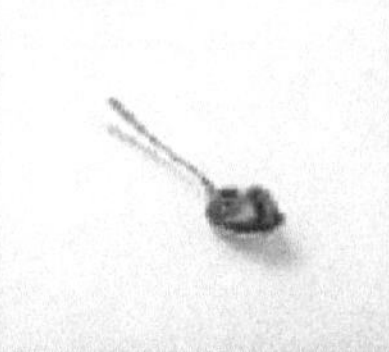	**Spirits (ABV 40%)** One measure or 'shot' (25ml) 56 kcal 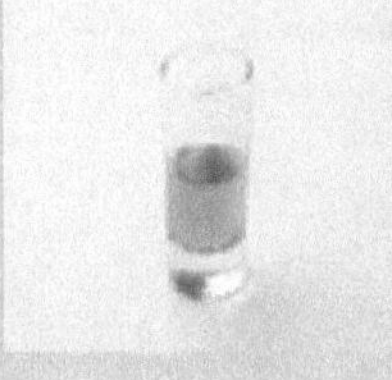	**Chocolate** Three squares 78 kcal 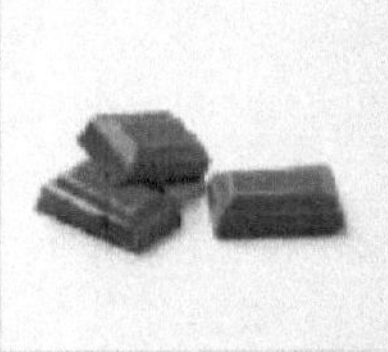
Biscuits, plain Two 100 kcal 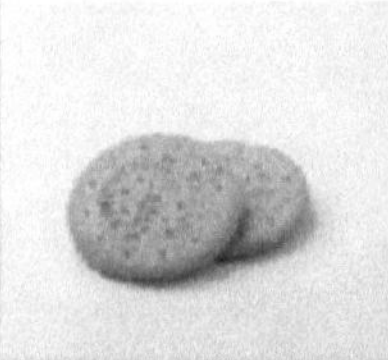	**Sweets** One small tube or bag 90 kcal 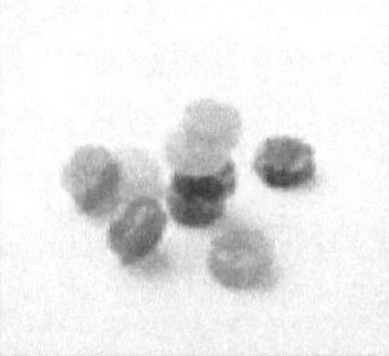	**Glass of wine (ABV 12%)** One small glass (125ml) 100 kcal 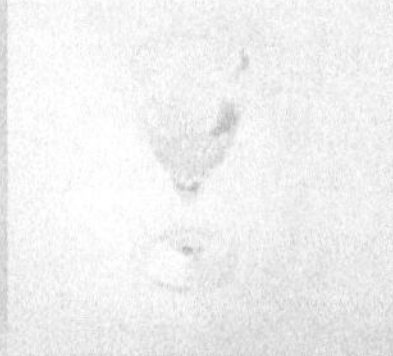	**Ice cream** One small scoop 100 kcal 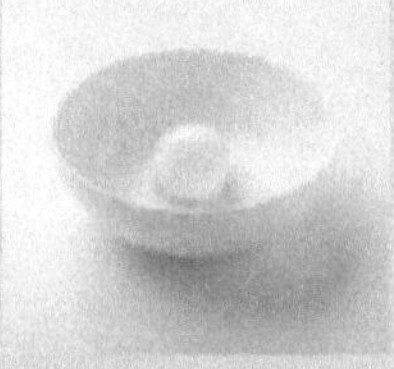
Lager, cider or beer (ABV 5%) Half pint 117 kcal 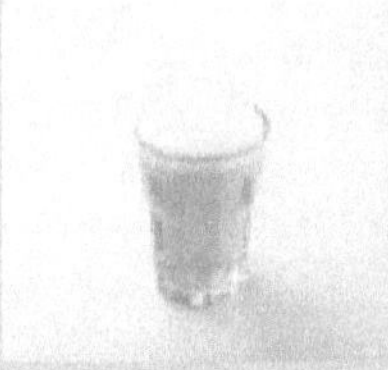	**Bottle of beer (ABV 5%)** One 330ml bottle 135 kcal 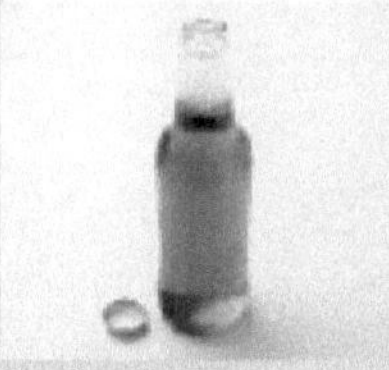	**Slice of cake** One small slice (50g) 150 kcal 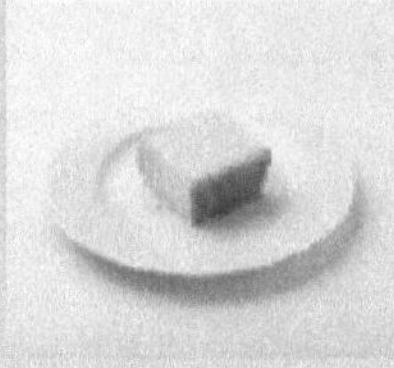	**Crisps** One small packet (25g) 150 kcal 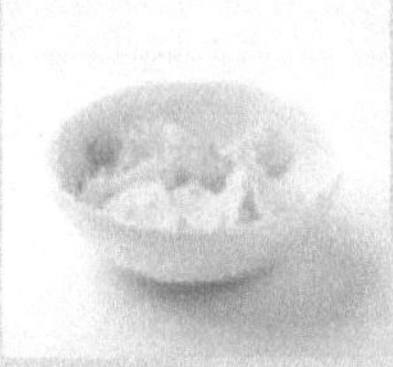

Mini pork pie	Quiche/tart	Chocolate bar	Danish pastry
One 196 kcal	One quarter of a small (60g) 250 kcal	One bar (45g) 240 kcal	Danish pastry (110g) 376 kcal

Tips for eating less fatty and sugary foods

- Choose 'diet', no added sugar or unsweetened versions of fizzy drinks, squashes and fruit juice

- Instead of snacks such as crisps, chocolate, pakora, samosas, sweet pastries and biscuits – choose fruit, plain popcorn, wholegrain crackers or raw vegetables with a low fat dip like salsa or cucumber and yoghurt

- Use semi skimmed milk, 1% or skimmed milk rather than condensed milk or coconut milk.

Alcohol , calories and your health

Alcoholic drinks are included in this group. Most people enjoy a drink or two and there's no reason why you shouldn't have an
occasional drink when you're trying to lose weight. But alcohol is
high in sugar, so it's high in calories too – drinks can really add up
and affect your weight loss. Also, because alcohol is an appetite

stimulant, some people notice they tend to eat more when they
drink alcohol.

This table shows you the amount of calories in some common drinks:			
Drink	**Units**	**Calories (kcal)**	**Same as...**
25ml single spirit (ABV 40%)	1 Unit	56	3 fancy filled individual chocolates (66 kcal)
50ml of cream liqueur (ABV 17%)	1 Unit	118	Slice of Battenberg cake (119 kcal)
275ml bottle of alcopop (ABV 5.5%)	1.5 Units	170	2 chocolate covered biscuits (178 kcal)
330ml bottle of strong lager, beer or cider (ABV 5%)	1.6 Units	135	25g pack of salted crisps (132 kcal)
440ml can of regular lager, beer or cider (ABV 4.5%)	2.6 Units	182	Slice of sponge cake with cream and jam (182 kcal)
Standard glass (175ml) of red, white or rosé wine (ABV 13%)	2.3 Units	166	37g tube of chocolate covered sweets (169 kcal)
Standard glass (125ml) champagne (ABV 12%)	1 Unit	86	9 sweets (90 kcal)
Pint of strong lager, beer or cider (ABV 5%)	2.8 Units	233	Sugar doughnut (242 kcal)
Large glass (250ml) of red, white or rosé wine (ABV 13%)	3.3 Units	195	Mini pork pie (196 kcal)
Pint of extra strong lager, beer or cider (ABV 8%)	4.5 Units	358	Medium takeaway chicken curry (377 kcal)
Bottle (750ml) of red, white or rosé wine (ABV 13.5%)	10 Units	712	2 shish kebabs (714 kcal)

Drinking too much alcohol can also be harmful to your health. It can lead to muscle damage, high blood pressure, stroke and some cancers. So if you drink alcohol, it's important to keep within the sensible limits, however often you drink.

Know your units

A unit is a measure of alcohol. The number of units is based on
the size of the drink and its alcohol strength. The ABV (alcohol by
volume) figure is the percentage of alcohol in the drink. Different
strengths of drinks can contain different amounts of alcohol.

1 unit of alcohol =			
One single pub measure (25ml) of spirits (ABV 40%)	One half pint (about 300ml) of normal-strength lager, cider or beer (ABV 3.5%)	(100ml) of wine (ABV 10%)	One glass (50ml) of liqueur, sherry or other fortified wine (ABV 20%)

Men	...should not regularly drink more than 3 to 4 units of alcohol in a day. That's not much more than a pint of strong lager, beer or cider.
Women	...should not regularly drink more than 2 to 3 units of alcohol in a day. That's no more than a standard 175ml glass of wine

Keep an eye on your glass size!
It's easier than you think for the units to add up when you're drinking wine or pouring your own drinks. Note that wine is only 100ml for a unit, but normal sizes for glasses of wine in the pub are either 175ml (small) or 250ml (large) so that means a glass will be more than one unit.

Think about drinks

Drinking enough is an important part of keeping healthy so you
need to have regular non-alcoholic drinks – around 6 to 8 drinks

a day.
The amount of drink you need does vary though – for example if
you do more activity than usual or if it's a hot day you will need to
drink more. You will get some water from the food you eat, but you
still need to drink too.
Many people don't realise how many calories they take in through
their drinks, so when looking over your food diary think about
what you drink and what swaps you can make.

Cold drinks

Water is the best choice, but you can include other non-alcoholic
drinks during the day such as sugar-free squash or fruit juice.
Avoid fizzy drinks that contain a lot of sugar and calories so choose
sugar-free or 'diet' alternatives instead. Flavoured waters with a
hint of fruit are also good for mixing it up, but check they don't
have any added sugar.

Hot drinks

You can include some tea and coffee among your daily drinks,
but it's important that this isn't your only source of fluid. This is
because they make it harder for your body to absorb the iron you

need from the food you eat and also contain caffeine, which is
a stimulant.
If you add sugar to your tea and coffee, try gradually reducing the
amount you have by half a teaspoon so you get used to the taste
before cutting it out completely. Remember to also think about
the amount of milk in hot drinks as this can add calories – at home
or in the coffee shop go for the skinny option (using skimmed milk) and skip the cream on hot chocolate.

Alcoholic drinks

Alcoholic drinks should be counted as part of the foods high in fat and/or sugar group. See page 68 for more details.

'M y top tip is to drink
plenty of water.
It's the best drink
you can have when
you're losing weight
because it's got
no sugars in it,
and no calories.'
Rif lost 13lbs

Eating plan

To the right is an example eating plan which shows food and drink choices for both 1,500 and 1,800 kcal.

Obviously no two days are the same and not all of these options may suit you, but it shows you how the plan works and the range of foods you could eat.

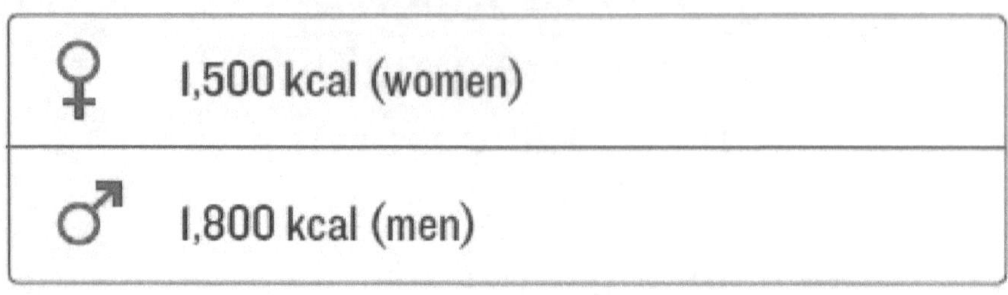

Meals

Your weight loss plan will mean making changes, but that doesn't
mean you have to stop eating your favourite meals. Nor does it
mean you have to spend hours in the kitchen preparing special
foods. In fact, many healthy and tasty meals are easy to prepare.
If you want to try some new and exciting meals, sign up to our free
Heart Matters service. You will be able to access our online recipe
finder to search over 140 delicious heart healthy recipes and watch
cooking videos of some of our favourites. You will also receive our
Heart Matters magazine, which is full of great meal ideas.
Go to **bhf.org.uk/heartmatters** to find out more.

*BHF / heart matters recipes		**Food Group**					
Meals		Fruit and veg	Bread, rice, potato	Milk and dairy	Meat, fish, eggs	Spreading fats, oils & dressing	Foods and drinks high in fat and sugar
For 1500 kcal	Number of portions	5+	7	3	2	2	
For 1800 kcal	Number of portions	5+	8	3	3	2	
Breakfast							
Shredded Wheat			2				
Semi skimmed milk	200ml			1			
Glass fruit juice	150ml	1					
Tea, milk no sugar							
Toast wholegrain			1				
Low fat spread	1tsp					½	
Jam	2 tsp						50 kcal
Mid-morning							
Tea							
Apple		1					
Lunch							
Egg and tomato wrap*							
Wrap	1		2				
Boiled egg	2				1		
Low fat cheese	2 tbs			1			
Tomato	1	½					
Lettuce							
Side salad	1 bowl	1					
Water							
Malt loaf	1 slice 35g		1				

Dinner

Spaghetti bolognaise

		Fruit and veg	Bread, rice, potato	Milk and dairy	Meat, fish, eggs	Spreading fats, oils & dressing	Foods and drinks high in fat and sugar
Spaghetti*	6 heaped tbs		2				
Meat sauce* Made with tinned tomatoes, onion, carrots, celery and mushrooms	⅛ ¼	1			1 2		
Mixed green salad		1					
Fat free dressing	2 tbs					1	
Yoghurt	200g			1			
Glass wine	125ml						100 kcal
Total	1500 kcal	5 ½	7	3	2	1	100 kcal
	1800 kcal	5 ½	8	3	3	1 ½	150 kcal

You can use the table below to track your portions

Meals	Food Group					
	Fruit and veg	Bread, rice, potato	Milk and dairy	Meat, fish, eggs	Spreading fats, oils & dressing	Foods and drinks high in fat and sugar
Breakfast						
Mid-morning						
Lunch						
Mid-afternoon						
Dinner						
Total						

REMEMBER! You don't have to use all your allowance on one day – you can balance it out over the week to make it work for you. There are two more of these tables at the back of this booklet, and you can also download and print more tracking sheets from bhf.org.uk/factsnotfads

Cutting down on salt and saturated fat

To keep your heart healthy it's important that you don't eat too
much salt or saturated fat.
Eating too much salt can increase your risk of high blood pressure,
and this increases your chance of developing coronary heart disease. The recommended maximum amount of salt for adults
is 6g a day – which is about a level teaspoon. Most people don't
realise how much salt they're having and go over this limit
Remember that all types of salt count including sea salt, flakes,
crystals and garlic salt and it's not just about the salt that you add
to food yourself. Most of the salt we eat is 'hidden' in foods. Foods

high in salt include soups, sauces, cheese, savoury snacks, biscuits,
pizza, ready meals and fast foods. There can also be a lot of salt
in everyday foods like bread and breakfast cereals.

'I think you should be able to give
yourself treats. The weekend is
a natural time to 'go wild', so I do –
but not that wild!'
Andy lost 1st 7lbs

Top tips for reducing your salt intake

- Add less salt when cooking – don't use it when you're boiling vegetables or pasta for example.

- Don't add salt to your food at the table – your taste buds will soon adapt to the taste. Experiment with herbs and spices to add extra flavour.

- Choose foods labelled 'low salt' or 'no added salt'.

- Swap salty snacks such as crisps and salted nuts for fruit and vegetables.

- Avoid saltier foods such as bacon, cheese, takeaways, ready meals and other processed food.

Saturated fats

These can raise the amount of cholesterol in your blood, especially the harmful LDL cholesterol which increases the risk of fatty deposits developing in your arteries.

Top tips to cut the amount of fat you eat

- Cut down on high fat snacks like crisps, chocolates, biscuits, samosas and pakoras.

- Change to low fat dairy products: use semi-skimmed or skimmed milk and choose low fat yoghurts and cheese.

- Buy the leanest cuts of meat you can and avoid processed meat products like sausages and bacon.

- Remove the skin and visible fat from meat before cooking.

- Try baking, boiling, steaming, poaching or microwaving your food instead of frying, so that you don't need to add fat. Buy a non-stick frying pan and roasting tray so you can cook without adding fat.

- Measure out oil with a teaspoon or use spray oil rather than pouring it straight from the bottle.

- Spoon off fats and oils from casseroles and curries.

Food labels

Getting to grips with food labels will help you compare
products
when you're shopping and make healthier choices to support
your
weight loss.
Most foods have a nutritional information panel either on the
back
or side of the pack. Find the 'per 100g' column, and then
compare
them with the figures shown in the box below to see whether
it's
low, medium or high.

All measures per 100g	Low A healthier choice	Medium OK most of the time	High Just occasionally	
Sugars	5g or less	5.1g – 22.5g	More than 22.5g	More than 27g/portion
Fat	3g or less	3.1g – 17.5g	More than 17.5g	More than 21g/portion
Saturates	1.5g or less	1.6g – 5g	More than 5g	More than 6g/portion
Salt	0.30g or less	0.31g – 1.5g	More than 1.5g	More than 1.8g/portion

As well as looking at labels, here are a few more tips for successful
food shopping:
• Write a list before you go – this will help you focus only on what
you need and could save you time and money too.
• Never go shopping when you're hungry – you'll find it much easier to avoid temptation and just buy the foods you'd planned.
• Get smart about 'bargains' – we all love to save money, but if the
special offers are on foods high in calories is it really worth it?

<u>*Eating out*</u>

Eating out usually means we have little control over how food is
prepared or how large the portion is. The food also tends to be
high in fat, salt and sugar and the healthy choices are not that
obvious. But there are some things you can do to reduce the
impact on your weight loss goals, meaning having the odd meal
out is unlikely to make a difference to your weight in the long
run.

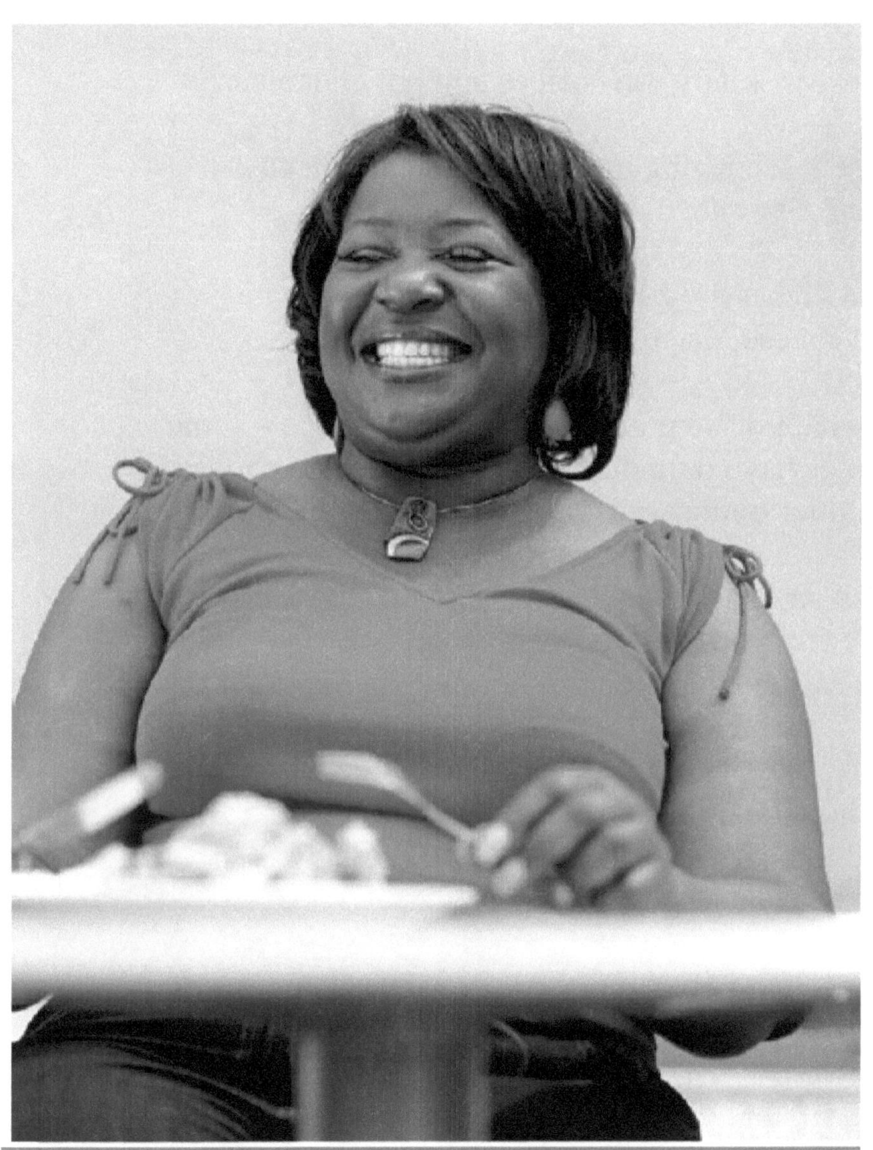

Top tips:

• Ask to go 'skinny' on coffees and hot chocolate.

• Choose a scone or currant bun instead of a pastry,
cream cake or chocolate muffin.

• If sandwiches are being made deli style, say no
to extra cheese, mayo and sauces.

• Plan what you're going to eat before you go – some
companies have online menus you can use to choose
the healthier options.

• Portion sizes are often bigger when you're eating out
so don't feel you have to finish what's on your plate.
Share a starter or pudding rather than having your own.

• Ask for dressings and sauces on the side so you can
decide how much to add and remember the 'extras'
you add like cheese, sour cream and dressings can
be high in fat and salt.

• Go for tomato or vegetable-based sauces and soups
rather than cream, coconut or cheese-based ones.

• Choose plain boiled rice instead of fried and go for
boiled or jacket potatoes rather than chips or wedges.

• Choose steamed or stir-fried options rather than
deep-fried dishes – batter is off the menu!

<u>**SECTION 4: Strategies for success**</u>

'T he hardest part about losing weight is the time it takes – it's not overnight. My advice is to focus on yourself, make small goals and take realistic baby steps.'
Emma lost 9st

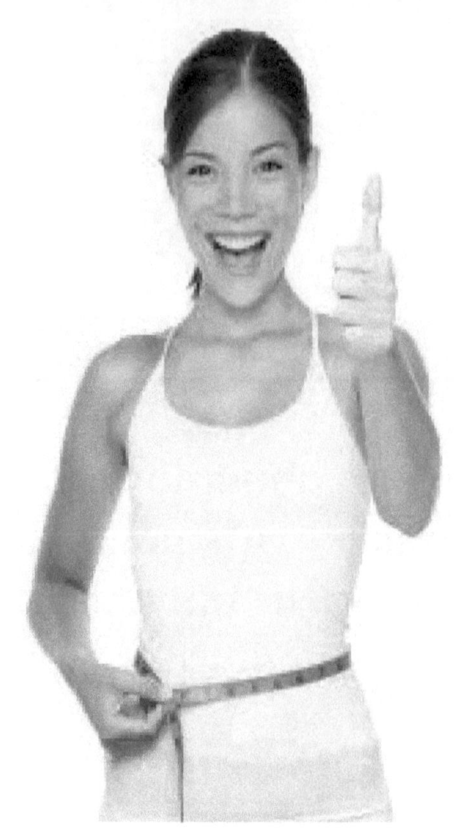

<u>*Stay on track*</u>

• Think positive: Rather than concentrating on what
you can't have, focus on ways to eat more healthily.

• Overcome obstacles with forward planning: Think
how you will deal with challenging situations before
they arise. For instance, if you are eating out you can
check the menus beforehand to find a healthy option.

• Identify changes: Look over your goals and pick out
what you need to do to achieve them or who might
be able to help. For example, talking to your family,
clearing out your cupboards, looking up some recipes
or asking a friend at work to join you in lunchtime walks.

• Don't let one slip ruin your hard work – a lapse is not
a collapse. If you break your plan for a few hours or
days, it is not the end of the world. Try not to see your
goals as 'all or nothing'. Learn from what went wrong
and get back on track as soon as you are ready.

• Make sure you plan something (healthy) to reward
yourself when you reach your goals (see page 89) –
this will keep you going if it does get tough.

<u>*Make small changes*</u>

Start small. Small changes add up to a big difference and they
don't need to be difficult.

Small change	Calories (kcal) saved
Leaving off the spread from a sandwich	57
Swap your croissant for a wholemeal fruit scone	60
Swap a chocolate covered biscuit for an apple	73
Swap a pint of semi skimmed milk for skimmed	79
Instead of cheese (40g) on toast go for beans (80g)	101
Switching a can of fizzy drink to sugar free squash	127

For heart healthy recipes, sign up to our free Heart Matters service.
You'll be able to access our online recipe finder and also receive
our Heart Matters magazine which is full of great meal ideas.
You can also download our Healthy Heart Recipe Finder app to
your iPhone or Android smartphone. It has over 100 recipes from
all over the world and a handy shopping list feature.
Go to **bhf.org.uk/heartmatters** to find out more.

'I try to focus on the real benefit for me, and what makes me feel good. I think that's the key thing.'
Pam lost 3st

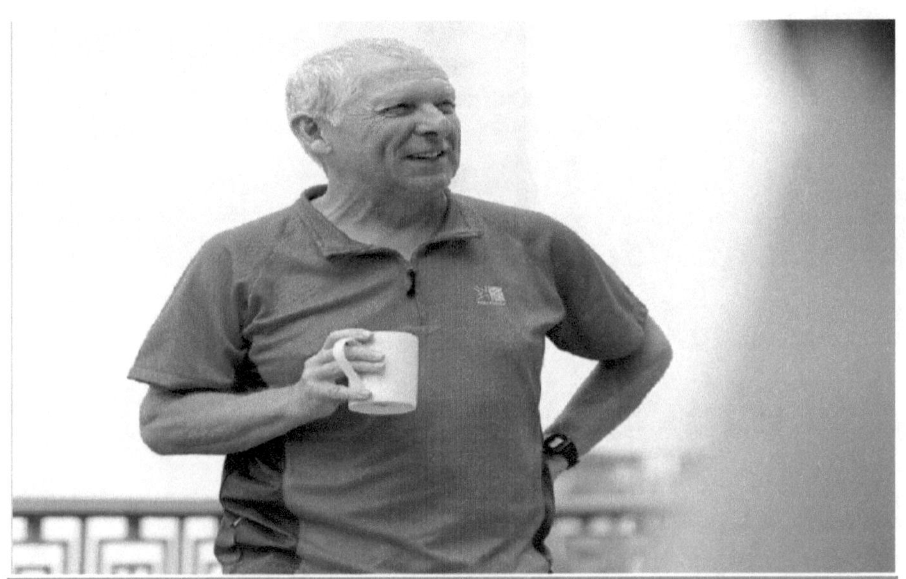

Change your behaviour

As you know, changing your diet needs a lot of careful thought
and effort. Often we know what we should be doing, but
somehow find it difficult to stick to changes. That's not to say it's
always an uphill battle, but there are some things you can do to

make it a bit easier for yourself. Many of these things involve a little
planning ahead or thinking about things differently. They all help
you feel more in control of what you are trying to achieve.
For a lot of people these 'behaviour changes' are the key to successful and permanent weight loss.

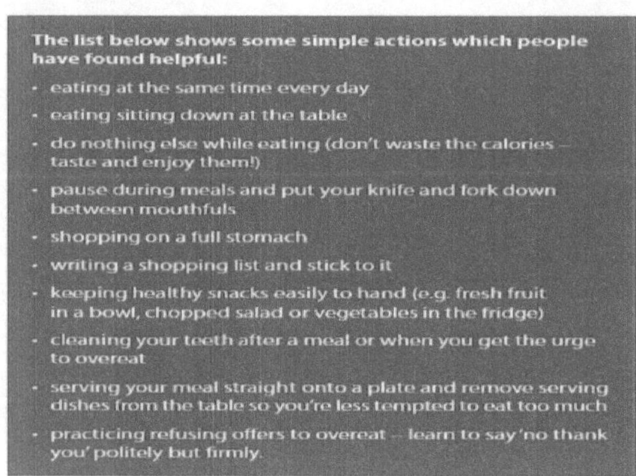

The list below shows some simple actions which people have found helpful:

- eating at the same time every day
- eating sitting down at the table
- do nothing else while eating (don't waste the calories — taste and enjoy them!)
- pause during meals and put your knife and fork down between mouthfuls
- shopping on a full stomach
- writing a shopping list and stick to it
- keeping healthy snacks easily to hand (e.g. fresh fruit in a bowl, chopped salad or vegetables in the fridge)
- cleaning your teeth after a meal or when you get the urge to overeat
- serving your meal straight onto a plate and remove serving dishes from the table so you're less tempted to eat too much
- practicing refusing offers to overeat — learn to say 'no thank you' politely but firmly.

Know your danger points

As well as things you can do differently, there are also ways you
can teach yourself to think differently. Along with your food diary,
using the suggestions below can help you get your 'mind over
matter' and feel more in control of your weight loss.

Real hunger or cravings

A regular eating pattern is the best way to keep hunger at bay,

but often you can experience a strong urge to eat, usually for a
specific type of food such as a pudding after a very filling evening
meal. Before you eat, check that you are really hungry rather than
just eating at a certain time or occasion out of habit. Try waiting
20 minutes, if you aren't actually hungry these feelings will pass.
Using distractions will also help you control your eating – make
a phone call, do the washing up or clean your teeth.

Feelings or triggers

Be aware of how your feelings affect what you want to eat.
For example do you eat more when you are bored, lonely or upset?
Noticing a pattern can help you plan how to cope. Identifying
activities apart from food that you find comforting is one way
round this problem. You could treat yourself to a new magazine
or listen to your favourite music instead.

Reward yourself

Rewards can make it more likely you will achieve your goals.
They should not be food or drink and need not be expensive.
Here are some suggestions that have worked for others:
• time to yourself such as a soak in the bath or sitting in
the garden
• buy yourself a new magazine, item of make up, new DVD
or video game

- take a trip to a cinema, theatre or art gallery

- have a manicure, pedicure or massage

- donate to your favourite charity.

<u>*EMMA's story*</u>

I knew I was really overweight, but I didn't want to
acknowledge it, so I just sort of forgot about it. But I got
to a place where I knew if I got any bigger I would never
be happy unless I started losing weight.

My friend is a personal trainer and she offered to help me, but
because of an existing illness she said I needed go to the
doctor
to get checked out before we started. I went and they gave
me
the BHF weight loss plan to do alongside the exercise.
I went home and read the plan and said 'right this is it – it's
now
or never'. So although I'd put on the weight gradually the
decision
to start losing weight was an overnight thing – everything
had
clicked into place.
The hardest part about losing weight is the time it takes – it's
not
overnight. I've lost nearly 9 stone now and sometimes it was
hard
to keep it going. But there's no way of getting round it – no
weight
loss is easy. And I know that I'm always going to have to
watch

what I eat.
Starting cycling really helped me. I set myself the goal of
completing the BHF London to Brighton bike ride. My first 6 miles
of training were awful – I hated every minute of it, puffing and
panting. But after a while I started to really enjoy it. Now I can cycle
75 miles plus with no problem, it's become a social thing and my
boyfriend and I go out for a ride as much as we can. We get to
spend time together and it's so much better for me than sitting
in a pub or on the sofa thinking about what I can eat.

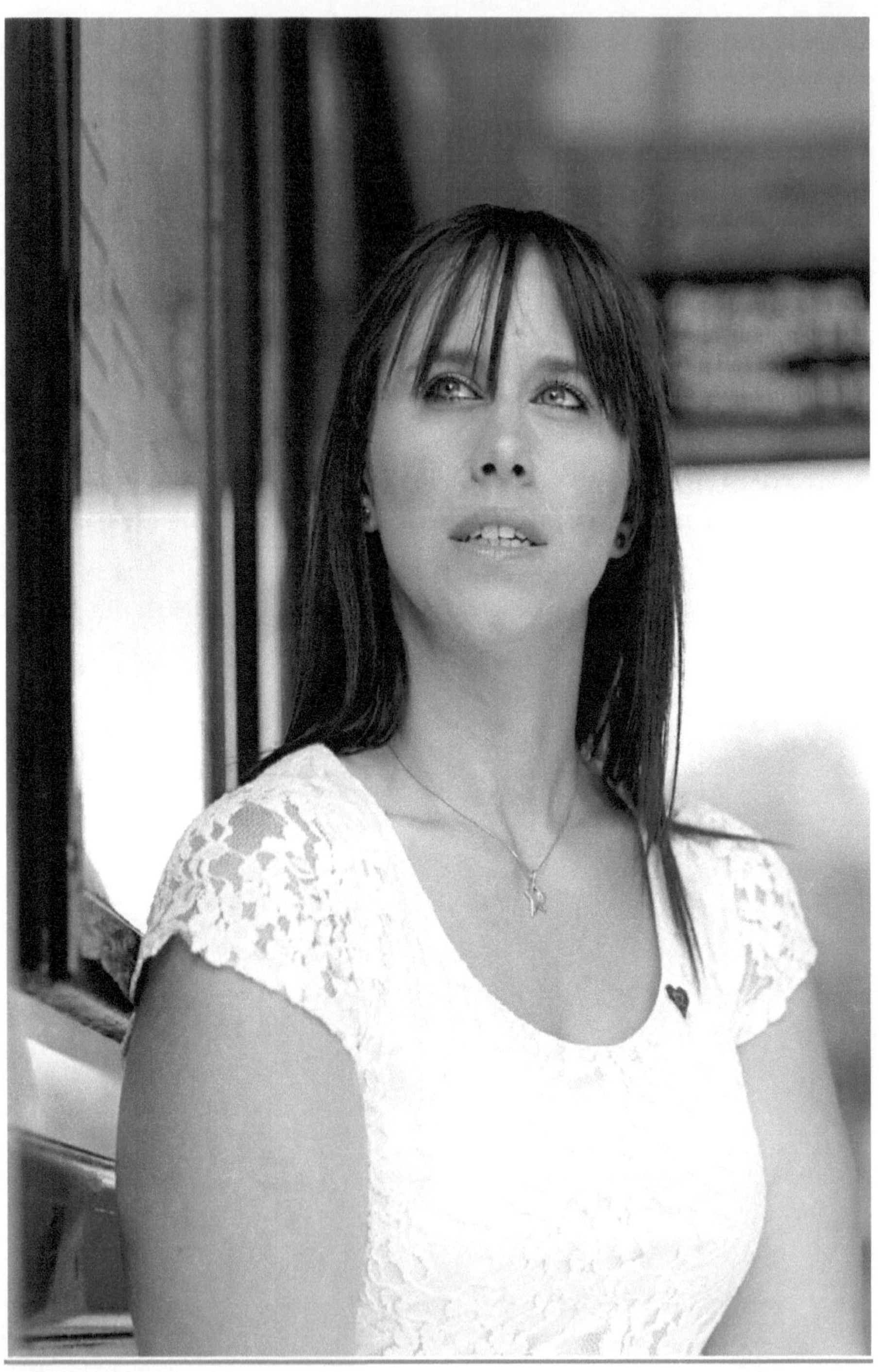

<u>**Get moving**</u>

This guide has mainly focused on how to reduce your calorie
intake to help you lose weight, but you will know from page
14
that you can also lose weight by increasing the amount of
calories
you burn being active. Increasing your daily activity helps
burn
calories that would otherwise end up stored as fat. It also
builds
muscle. The more muscle you have the more energy your
body
uses when resting and the easier it is to lose weight.
Regular activity is a vital part of your weight loss journey – it's
essential to maintain a healthy weight in the long term.
Physical
activity also improves your heart health and reduces the risk
of
developing heart disease, diabetes and some cancers. This is
true
no matter what weight you are or how much weight you lose
as
a result of being active.

Physical activity	Calories Burnt	
	Based on 40 year old weighing 11 stone (70kg)	Based on 60 year old weighing 14 stone (89kg)
10 mins walking up stairs	93	135
30 mins washing the car	157	229
30 mins mowing the lawn	192	279
30 mins of ironing	80	117
1 hour of golf	314	457
1 hour of light dog walking	196	284
30 mins light rowing machine	122	178
30 mins medium swimming	279	406
30 mins recreational badminton	314	457
30 mins medium walking	175	254
30 mins medium cycling	279	406

How much should you aim to do?

For weight loss and heart health, you should aim to exercise daily and in total should be clocking up at least 150 minutes of moderate intensity activity every week – that's activity which
involves moving different parts of your body, getting slightly breathless (but still able to talk) and becoming a little hot and sweaty.

This doesn't have to mean going to classes or taking up jogging.
It's more about finding something which suits you – and which is
safe and enjoyable. Aim to increase your activity levels gradually.
Start by aiming for up to half an hour a day of moderate activity
on at least five days of the week. Then build this up gradually to
help with your weight loss.

<u>What activity should you do?</u>

You can build activity into your everyday life with a bit of thought
and determination. Walking is particularly good because it doesn't
cost anything and you don't need a membership or any special
kit other than sensible shoes! People have found that taking the
stairs instead of the lift (up as well as down), walking to the shops,
cycling to work, digging the garden or playing outdoors with the
children can make quite a difference.
If more structured exercise appeals to you – such as swimming,
the gym or exercise classes – find out if your local leisure centre
runs sessions at a time which suits you.
Our **Get active, stay active** booklet has information, tips and

support to help you set some goals and build activity into your
day – download or order for free at **bhf.org.uk/publications**.
If you have any health problems, check with your doctor before
starting a physical activity programme.
We also have an online physical activity calculator which is easy
to use and a great way to see how all activity counts towards
your weight loss – from daily chores to more intense activity like
running or cycling. The table shows some examples, but go to
bhf.org.uk/calories to get the results tailored to you.

SECTION 5:

track your progress

'I think you've got to choose something you enjoy, research it, and stick to it. To sustain it you need to be able to give yourself little rewards from time to time.'
Andy lost 1st 7 lbs

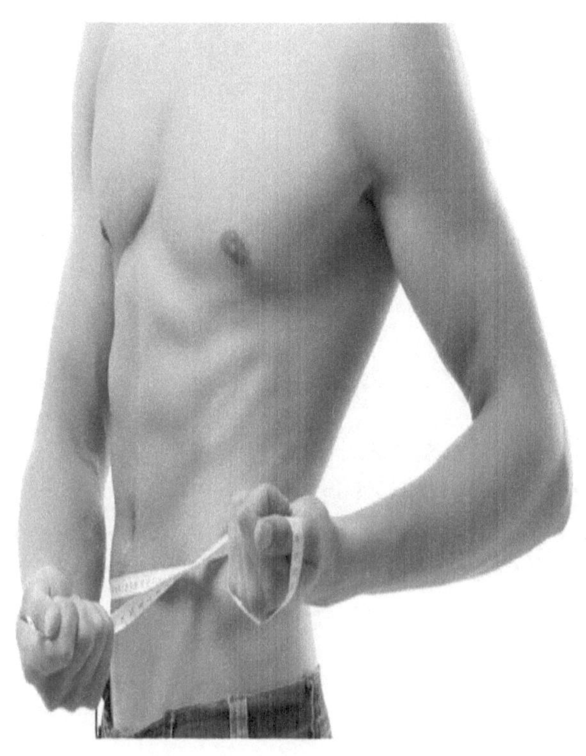

TRACK YOUR PROGRESS

It's really important to track your progress so you can see how
you are doing and check your progress against the S.M.A.R.T.
goals you have set yourself. The chart on page 100 will help

you to record everything.

<u>Monitoring your weight</u>

We recommend you keep a regular record of your weight.
But don't be tempted to weigh yourself more than once a
week.
Weigh yourself on the same scales and at the same time of
day,
without clothes if possible. Remember you are looking for a
gradual weight loss of 1-2 pounds (0.5-1 kg) per week.
There may be some weeks when you lose more weight than
this
and other weeks where your weight may stay the same or go
up. There can be many reasons for this – being unwell, a
special
occasion, water retention or being more active – but by
tracing
everything you will be able to look back and see why this may
have happened.

Rewards

Make sure you plan your non-food-based rewards (see page
89)
to keep you going when it gets tough, and to give yourself a
pat
on the back when you get there. You can use them for
reaching
'behaviour' goals as well as weight goals. Make sure you think
about how you are going to reward yourself before you start
your weight loss plan, as this will motivate you.

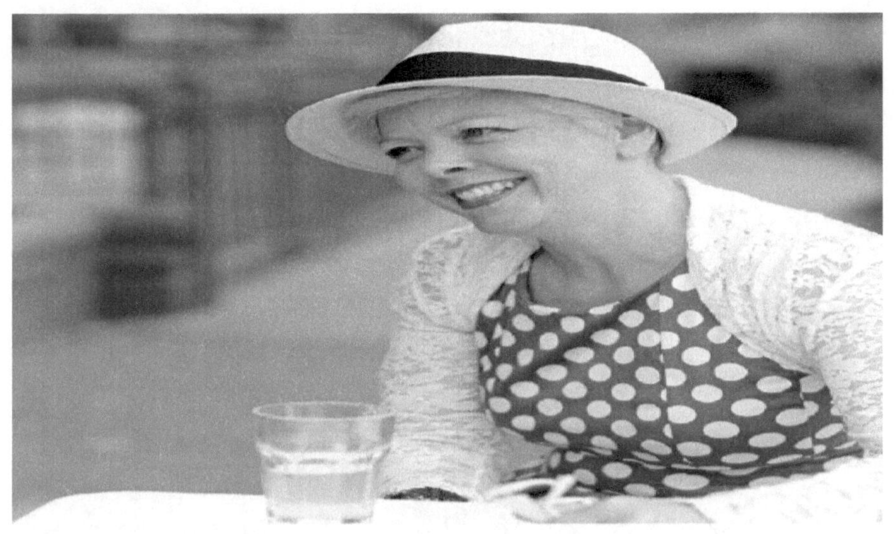

RIF'S STORY

My friends were the ones who encouraged me to lose
weight. They'd taken part in a weight loss programme
and I saw their results. One went seriously into it,
and now he looks younger and slimmer. If he can
do it I can do it as well.

I've started exercising twice a week. The main thing I've learnt
is
that you've got to keep going at it. In the past I would always
say
'I'm busy, I haven't got time'. I was always making excuses –
but
you can make time, you've got to put the effort in. You've just
got
to push yourself basically.
I've changed the way I'm eating. The hardest part was giving
up
the 'bad' foods, you know your children tend to like those
kind
of foods and it's temptation! But my advice would be to plan

your way in – I've found preparing food that was a lot healthier
does take more time, but if you have a menu ready for the week
it makes life a lot easier, so you go home, you know what you're
preparing, you've got the stuff there and ready for you.
I've lost just under a stone and 6cm from my waistline. It was quite
hard going – I've still got quite a way to go but it's quite a loss for me.
Now I'm fitting into trousers that I haven't worn for years – I feel
good that I'm back into some of my old jeans, and when a lot of
friends come up to you it boosts your confidence even more – all
those things have definitely encouraged me.
So I would say just don't give up, keep trying. If you keep going
you'll eventually succeed. A lot of people say 'I can't do it ' – but
there's no way you can if you don't try.

Rif lost 13lbs

Keep at it

Some people say losing weight is not that difficult,
it's keeping it off that's the hard bit!
If you have a tendency to gain weight, you'll always
need to keep an eye on your weight.

> **To keep to a healthy weight or to prevent weight gain:**
>
> - keep following the rules of the eatwell plate – you may
>   find that it becomes easier over time and that filling up on
>   foods from the main four food groups leaves you with less
>   space for the high-calorie 'fatty and sugary foods'
>
> - remind yourself how good it feels to have reached some
>   of your goals
>
> - if your weight goes up a bit, don't despair. By reassessing
>   things, making a few small changes, and getting support,
>   you will start to lose a few pounds again.

Pam'S STORY

I was about 15 years old when someone gave me a diet
book. At the time I didn't realise anyone thought of
me as overweight, and when I look back at pictures
I wasn't! But I started being conscious of what I ate.

From then on I yo-yo dieted, but a couple of years ago I made
a lasting change – I lost three stone and I've kept it off.
One of the key things was recognising how I feel and how that
affects how I eat. Thinking 'what do you really need? Do you need
a box of chocolates, or do you need to cry, or do you need a hug?'
For exercise what I've tried to do is find things that I really enjoy,
the stuff that I'd do even if there wasn't anyone cracking the whip.
I think you need to make sure you're going to the gym because you
want to feel good and you want to live longer and be healthier –
focus on the real benefit for you. That's the key thing.
One of the biggest challenges is other people's expectations –
'oh go on, treat yourself, live a little!' it's important to find ways
to feel strong in yourself, to not give in just because it's what
somebody else wants for you when it isn't what you want for you.
Concentrate on doing it because you're the one who wants to do

it and this is good for you.
I know I'm always going to have to have my eye on the ball. It can
sound a bit pessimistic but realistically I can't ever just say 'I'm not
going to think about how I feel or what I'm eating and now that
I'm thinner I can just live my life'. That's what I've done before and
I've just put the weight back on.
But there are definitely things about the way I eat and the way that
I feel and the way I react to things that I have changed for good.
I'm not forcing myself, it just that's the way I do it now. It's about
making habits that stick.
Pam lost 3st

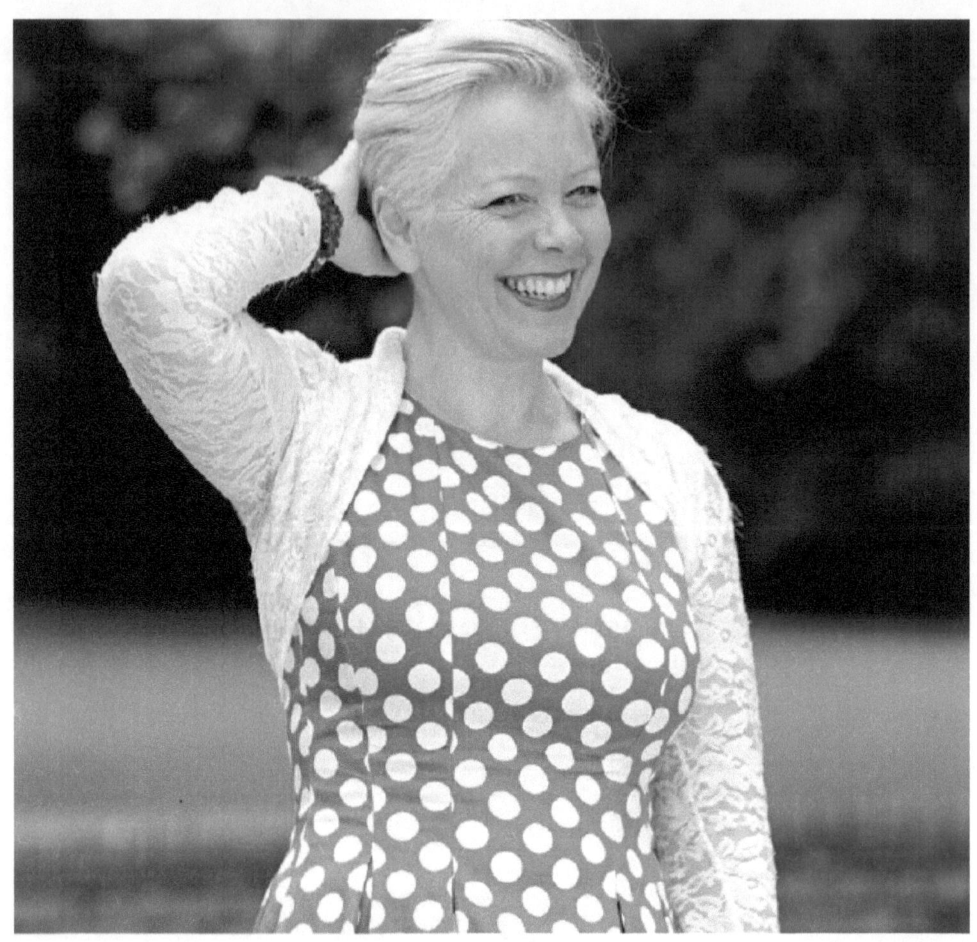

other options

If this weight loss plan isn't working for you, there are some
commercial and self-help alternatives available that meet best
practice guidelines and may suit you better.
If you need more personal, face to face support you may want
to join a commercial group such as Weight Watchers, Slimming
World or Counterweight. These may be available as weight loss
programmes on prescription in your area – talk to your doctor
about this.

There are also a number of online options – including the NHS
Choices 12 week weight loss plan.
If you do decide to try something different, make sure:
• the weight loss offered is realistic
• it provides complete nutrition (it doesn't miss any food groups out)
• it gives support and education
• you discuss it with a healthcare professional like your GP or a dietitian.

Need more help?

If you would like help from someone who can talk through your weight loss plan personally, ask your doctor to refer you to a dietitian, or talk to your practice nurse.